Your Pregnancy

QUESTIONS AND ANSWERS

Glade B Curtis is a Fellow of the American College of Obstetricians and Gynecologists. He has a private practice in Sandy, Utah, USA, dealing in obstetrics, gynaecology and infertility.

One of Dr Curtis's goals as a doctor is to provide patients with many types of information about the gynaecological and obstetric conditions they may have, problems they may encounter and procedures they may undergo. In pursuit of that goal, he has written this book as a companion to his best-selling book, *Your Pregnancy Week by Week*. He has also co-authored a book on gynaecological surgery.

Dr Curtis is a graduate of the University of Utah and the University of Rochester School of Medicine and Dentistry, Rochester, New York. He was an intern, resident and chief resident in Obstetrics and Gynecology at the University of Rochester Strong Memorial Hospital. He now has a very active private practice in Sandy, where he lives with his wife Debbie and their five children.

D F Hawkins is a Fellow of the Royal College of Obstetricians and Gynaecologists. He is an honorary consultant at Hammersmith Hospital in London and Emeritus Professor of Obstetric Therapeutics at the University of London. He is the consulting editor of *The Journal of Obstetrics and Gynaecology* and the author of numerous books and papers.

by the same author
Your Pregnancy Week by Week

Your Pregnancy

QUESTIONS AND ANSWERS

Glade B Curtis
MD FACOG

Consultant Editor
D F Hawkins
MD FRCOG

ELEMENT
Shaftesbury, Dorset • Rockport, Massachusetts
Brisbane, Queensland

Cover photograph courtesy of Zefa Stoehmarket
Cover design by The Bridgewater Book Company
Text design by Roger Lightfoot
Typeset by Bournemouth Colour Press
Printed and bound in Great Britain by
Creative Print and Design (Wales), Ebbw Vale

British Library Cataloguing in Publication
data available

Library of Congress Cataloging in Publication
data available

ISBN 1–85230–801–X

Note from the publisher
This book is in no way intended to replace, countermand or conflict with
the advice given to you by your own doctor. The ultimate decision
concerning care should be made between you and your medical practitioner.

Credit
The material on pp105–8 and 297–310 is copyright the Health Education
Authority, London, and is reproduced with their permission.

Contents

Acknowledgements   vi
Foreword   vii

Part I Before Pregnancy
1 Preparing for Pregnancy   3

Part II Your Pregnancy
2 Your Health and Medical Concerns   21
3 Tests on You and your Growing Baby   50
4 Medicines and Treatments for You   72
5 Nutrition, Exercise and Weight Management   80
6 Fatigue, Work and Pregnancy   99
7 More than One Baby!   109
8 Changes in your Growing Baby   116
9 Changes in You   129
10 Sex during Pregnancy   149
11 Your Partner and your Pregnancy   152
12 Sexually Transmitted Diseases   157
13 Substance Use and Abuse   164
14 Special Concerns of the Single Mother-to-be   171
15 Problems and Warning Signs   176
16 You should also Know   193

Part III The Birth of your Baby
17 Labour and Delivery   215

Part IV After your Baby is Born
18 After your Baby's Birth   251
19 Your New Baby   258
20 Feeding your Baby   269

Glossary   283
Useful Addresses   297
Index   311

Acknowledgements

━━

I have the honour of sharing in the joy, the excitement and even the heartbreak associated with the miracle of childbirth on a daily (and nightly) basis. I thank my patients and their families for allowing me to share in their experiences. I have answered many of these questions hundreds, if not thousands, of times, yet to the person asking the questions, the answer is critical.

My thanks to my wife, Debbie, and our family who have supported me in the pursuit of a profession that requires me to give a lot of time and energy to my patients. Their unfailing support, which is an inspiration to me, has continued during this and other projects. My thanks also to my parents for their endless love and support.

Judi Schuler's insight, persistence, commitment to excellence and accuracy continue to inspire and to challenge me. I appreciate her drive and ability to 'pull things together' and keep me focused.

Foreword

═══

I have endeavoured to include all the questions that have been posed to me (and other doctors I know) dealing with every aspect of pregnancy and childbirth. If you have any questions I haven't covered, which might be of interest to other pregnant women, I would appreciate your sending them to me care of the publisher, Element Books. If possible, I will include your question and my answer in subsequent editions.

Pregnancy is a special time in a woman's life – and an enjoyable one. By being informed and working with your doctor, you can provide your baby with the best possible start in life.

PART I

Before Pregnancy

CHAPTER 1

Preparing for Pregnancy

The other day I read about the '12 months of pregnancy'. Pregnancy only lasts for 9 months, doesn't it?
The actual length of a pregnancy (the growth of the fetus into a normal-sized baby) is only 9 months. What the author was referring to was the concept of *preparing for pregnancy*. The few months before you get pregnant can be as important as the 9 months the fetus develops inside your womb. Adding the two figures together gives you the concept of 12 months of pregnancy.

Why are these 3 or 4 months before pregnancy so important?
With good preparation your baby will get the best start it can towards a healthy life. These months give you time to prepare your body for conception and pregnancy. You can eat nutritiously, cut out alcohol and tobacco use, begin an exercise programme, get your weight under control and address other medical concerns such as diabetes or lupus.

What should I do to prepare for pregnancy?
You can do many things to prepare for pregnancy.

- Exercise regularly.
- Find out if the medicines you take on a regular basis can be decreased or discontinued. Ask your doctor if they are safe to take during pregnancy.
- Make sure your weight is under control. Pregnancy is not the time to lose weight.
- If you need X-rays or medical tests, get them done before trying to get pregnant.
- It's a good time to control or eliminate tobacco, alcohol or drug use.

. Decide where you want your baby delivered. Check if you have insurance cover.

Attention to these details *before* getting pregnant makes your pregnancy safer and more enjoyable.

Should I see my doctor before I get pregnant or wait until I am pregnant?

Seeing your doctor before you get pregnant helps you prepare for pregnancy. A visit before pregnancy clears up questions about any medicines you are taking. You can have a cervical smear and any other tests your doctor decides are necessary. You and your doctor can evaluate your current weight and set a target weight gain for a pregnancy. You will know you're in good health before getting pregnant; if you're not, you can make plans to get into the best shape you can before you become pregnant.

Are there laboratory tests I should have done before I get pregnant?

Your doctor may order a range of tests for you. These include:

. cervical smear
. rhesus factor test
. blood typing
. rubella titres

If you know you have other specific or chronic medical problems, such as diabetes, have these checked. If you have been exposed to hepatitis or Aids, tests should be done for these.

My last two pregnancies ended in miscarriages. Should I talk to my doctor before I get pregnant or can I wait until my pregnancy is confirmed?

The history of previous pregnancies can be very important in the success of your next pregnancy. It's true that in many situations nothing can be done to help or to avoid problems. The safest thing to do is talk to your doctor before you try to conceive. Tell your doctor what has happened in the past. Find out if there is anything you can do now or if there are risks with which you may have to deal.

Your Body in Pregnancy

I've heard that a woman's body becomes very different during pregnancy. What changes can I expect?
The changes your body goes through during pregnancy are incredible! Your breasts enlarge and the number of milk ducts to produce breast milk actually increases. Your organs become crowded by your enlarging uterus, which may cause you to urinate more often or give you heartburn or indigestion. You legs, feet and hands may swell. Your hair and skin often undergo changes. Compare the illustration on this page with that on page 130 to see how a woman's body changes in pregnancy.

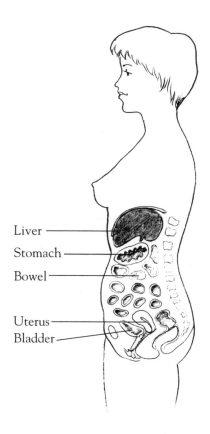

Liver
Stomach
Bowel

Uterus
Bladder

This illustration of a woman's body shows a non-pregnant uterus and various organs. Compare it with the one of a pregnant woman on page 130.

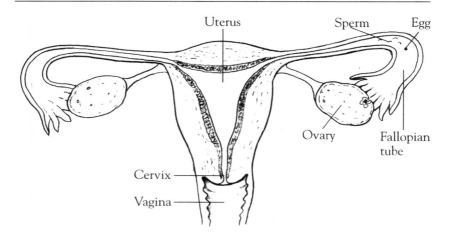

The miracle of pregnancy begins when the egg is fertilised by the sperm.

What is the purpose of the menstrual cycle?
During your menstrual cycle, your body prepares for the possibility of pregnancy. An egg is released from one of your ovaries, and changes take place in the lining of your uterus to provide an environment for the development of a fertilised egg. If fertilisation does not take place, the enriched lining is discarded through the menstrual flow.

I've heard that fertilisation is almost like a miracle. How does fertilisation of the egg occur?
Fertilisation is believed to occur in the middle part of the fallopian tube called the *ampulla*, not inside the uterus. Sperms travel through the uterine cavity and out into the tube to meet the egg (see the illustration above).

What happens after fertilisation?
The fertilised egg begins to divide and grow. Within 3 to 7 days, it travels down the tube into the uterus and attaches to the wall of the uterus. The developing baby is now often called an *embryo* (after 8 weeks it is usually called a *fetus*).

By about the 12th day, an amniotic sac begins to form around the developing embryo. The sac contains fluid in which the baby can easily move around. The amniotic fluid also cushions the fetus against injury and regulates temperature for it.

What is the 'bag of waters'?

This is another name for the membranes of the amniotic sac. When it is time for the baby to be born, these membranes must be broken so the birth can take place. If this does not happen naturally, the doctor or midwife will break them.

What is the placenta?

The placenta is a flat spongy structure that grows on the wall of the uterus and is attached to the baby by means of the umbilical cord.

What is the purpose of the placenta?

The placenta carries oxygen and nutrients from the mother to the fetus, and it carries carbon dioxide and waste products from the fetus to your body for excretion. It also produces hormones called *HCG* (*human chorionic gonadotropin*), *oestrogen* and *progesterone*.

What is an ectopic pregnancy?

An *ectopic pregnancy* is one in which the fertilised egg is implanted outside the uterus and starts to grow there. This is also called a *tubal pregnancy* because 95 per cent of the time it occurs in the fallopian tube. However, it may also happen in the ovary, the cervix or other locations in the abdomen. Because there is no way to nourish an embryo in these locations, an ectopic pregnancy must be ended (see illustration on page 183).

Where is the cervix?

The *cervix* is the necklike opening from the uterus into the vagina. Normally it is closed or very small (0.4in/1cm), and its tissue is firm and thick. It begins to enlarge, or dilate, when it is time for the baby to be born. It also becomes much softer, shorter and thinner, which is called *effacement*. The goal of labour is for it to become 100 per cent effaced and about 4in (10cm) dilated.

What is the birth canal?

The *birth canal* is the passage through which the baby travels to be born. It consists of the cervix, the vagina and the vulva.

Your Current Contraception Methods

If I want to get pregnant soon, when should I stop my birth control pills?
Most doctors recommend staying off the pill for two or three normal menstrual cycles before trying to get pregnant. Use some other form of contraception, such as a barrier method (condom), until you want to get pregnant.

How long should my coil be out before I try to conceive?
The best and easiest time to remove an IUCD is during your period. Wait for a couple of normal cycles after your IUCD is removed before trying to conceive. Use a barrier contraceptive during the waiting time.

I use Norplant for birth control. Is it all right to get pregnant immediately after it is taken out?
Once the Norplant is removed, wait at least two or three menstrual cycles before trying to get pregnant.

Your Pre-pregnancy Health

Can I have a successful pregnancy even though I have chronic health problems?
Yes. Most women with health problems have successful pregnancies and healthy babies. It is very important for you to discuss your particular situation with your doctor *before* becoming pregnant. Follow his or her instructions carefully.

I have diabetes, and I really want to have a baby. Is it possible?
Diabetes can have serious effects during pregnancy. Risks to you and your baby can be decreased with good control of blood sugar or control of your diabetes before and during pregnancy. Discuss your concerns with your physician *before* you try to conceive.

How long must the diabetes be under good control before I get pregnant?
Most doctors recommend 2 or 3 months before pregnancy begins. This helps lower the risk of miscarriage or of the fetal development being affected.

Will pregnancy affect my insulin requirements?
It can. Pregnancy can increase your body's need for insulin.

When do most pregnancy problems occur for diabetic women?
Most problems occur during the first trimester – the first 13 weeks of pregnancy. However, problems can occur throughout pregnancy. This is one important reason to have your diabetes under good control for 3 or 4 months before you conceive. It is also important to note that the mother's insulin requirement usually increases in the last 13 weeks of pregnancy.

I have asthma. Will pregnancy affect me?
There is no way to predict how your pregnancy will affect your asthma. About 50 per cent of those women affected see no change in their asthma during pregnancy. About 25 per cent have improved symptoms, while 25 per cent have increased problems.

Is my asthma medicine safe to take during pregnancy?
Most medicines prescribed for asthma are safe to use during pregnancy. Discuss your medicines with your doctor.

Is there anything else I can do to avoid asthma problems?
Avoid whatever substances trigger your asthma attacks.

I have high blood pressure, and I want to get pregnant. What kind of problems might I expect during pregnancy?
High blood pressure can cause problems for the mother and the baby. These include kidney damage, stroke or headaches in the mother-to-be and decreased blood flow to the fetus. The decreased blood flow can cause intra-uterine growth retardation (inadequate growth of the fetus).

Can I continue my blood-pressure medicine during pregnancy?
Some medicines are safe to take during pregnancy; others are not. Do *not* stop or decrease any medicines on your own! Discuss your situation with your doctor.

I've had heart problems for quite a while, but I want to have a baby. Is this dangerous?
Some heart problems may be serious during pregnancy and require special care. Other heart problems may affect your health so adversely

that your doctor will advise against pregnancy. This serious question must be discussed with your heart specialist and your obstetrician before your make any decision.

I have lupus, and with my first flare-up my kidneys were affected. Is this a serious consideration before I get pregnant?
Any situation that results in loss of kidney function can be serious during pregnancy. Be sure your doctor knows about this situation before you get pregnant. You will need to make a plan to follow during your pregnancy.

My mother always warned me not to try to have a baby because I have epilepsy. Should I avoid pregnancy?
I cannot answer this question without knowing your full medical history. I can tell you that some seizure medicines are safe to take during pregnancy, and nearly all women with epilepsy have successful pregnancies.

What kind of problems can I expect if I have epilepsy?
Mothers with epilepsy have a 1-in-30 chance of having a baby with a seizure disorder. Babies also have a higher incidence of birth defects, but this can be largely prevented by taking folic acid supplements, starting before conception. Seizures can be dangerous for you and your developing fetus, so it is extremely important for you to take your medicine as prescribed before and during pregnancy.

What kind of seizure medicine is safest to take during pregnancy?
Research has shown that phenobarbitone is fairly safe to take before and during pregnancy. Discuss its use with your physician, but do *not* discontinue or decrease your medicine on your own!

I've been told I was anaemic in the past. Should I start taking iron now?
Anaemia can be easily checked by your doctor. When you're pregnant, there are great demands on your body's iron supplies for the baby. Many women start taking vitamins or iron before getting pregnant. Because you have had a problem in the past, it's better to discuss this with your doctor before pregnancy.

I've heard there's a new drug being used for sickle cell anaemia, which I have. Can I use it while I try to get pregnant?
You are probably referring to *hydroxyurea*, which has proved to be the first effective treatment of sickle cell anaemia. It helps reduce the excruciating pain of some sickle cell attacks, but its use carries some risk and it cannot be given to all sickle cell sufferers. Because the use of the drug is so new, no one yet knows the possible adverse effects on the developing fetus or the long-term effects, so women who are contemplating pregnancy are advised *not* to use it.

I take thyroid medicine for a thyroid problem. Do I need to change the dose or stop taking it if I want to get pregnant?
Don't make *any* changes without first consulting your doctor. Medicine for thyroid problems is very important during pregnancy.

Will an occasional bladder infection before pregnancy cause problems during pregnancy?
It shouldn't, so don't be alarmed if you have a bladder infection or a urinary tract infection (UTI) before or during pregnancy.

What about other health problems? Do I need to see my doctor about them before I get pregnant?
Yes, you should. It's best to have any chronic medical condition under control before you get pregnant. You will feel better, and it's better for your growing baby if you deal with these issues before pregnancy.

My friend had surgery for breast cancer a few months ago, and now she's talking about getting pregnant. Is that dangerous?
This is a very individual problem and depends on the seriousness of her cancer and the type of treatment your friend received. It is very important for your friend to talk to her doctor if she is thinking about getting pregnant and she is being treated for cancer. It is much easier and safer for the woman to make decisions about treatments or medicines before becoming pregnant than after.

I've been having a lot of back problems, and my orthopaedic surgeon wants to do some X-rays, a CT scan and an MRI. Should I have them before I get pregnant?
Yes, these tests should be completed before you consider conceiving. A good time to schedule these tests is right after the end of your period so you know you're not pregnant.

I just had a vaccination for rubella. Is it all right to stop my birth control and try to get pregnant?

No. Some vaccinations are safe during pregnancy and some are not. Most physicians believe it's wise to continue contraception for at least 3 months after receiving any type of vaccination.

I often have to take medicines for various problems. Can you give me some good advice about using medicines before pregnancy?

It's best to be cautious with your use of medicines while you are preparing for pregnancy and while you are trying to conceive. Follow these guidelines for safe use:

. Take all prescription medicines as they are prescribed.
. Do not use medicines you used in the past for current problems.
. Be careful with over-the-counter medicines. Many contain caffeine, alcohol and other additives.
. Never use anyone else's medicine for your medical problem.
. Notify your doctor immediately if you are using medicines and believe you might be pregnant.

I often take several vitamins and herbs. Can I continue to take them while I prepare for pregnancy?

It isn't a good idea to self-medicate with anything while preparing for or during your pregnancy. In excessive amounts certain vitamins, such as vitamin A, can increase the risk of birth defects. The key to vitamin use and nutrition during pregnancy is balance. A multivitamin preparation and folic acid are the only supplements most women need while they are trying to conceive.

I read somewhere that caffeine can make a woman infertile. Is that true?

Studies have shown that drinking 8 cups of coffee a day (1,600mg of caffeine) is associated with a decrease in a woman's fertility (ability to get pregnant). Some researchers think there is an association between excessive caffeine consumption and miscarriage.

Should I Consider Genetic Counselling?

My sister had a baby last year that was born with Down's syndrome.
I'm considering pregnancy. Should I have genetic counselling?
This is something to discuss with your doctor. The answer is based on
many factors, including your past health, your partner's health and
your family medical history.

What can genetic counselling tell me?
Genetic counselling won't give you an *exact* answer, but a counsellor
can discuss possibilities or probabilities regarding a planned pregnancy
and your baby. In a situation like the one you describe with your sister,
ask your doctor for advice.

Should everyone consider genetic counselling?
It is not necessary for every woman. If there is a family history of
problems, it is probably advisable to seek this type of counselling.
Other situations in which genetic counselling should be considered
include:

- women over 35
- when either you or your partner has a birth defect
- if you have delivered a baby with a birth defect
- if you have had three or more miscarriages in a row
- if you and your partner are related

Pregnancy for Older Couples

I'm 40 years old this month and want to have another baby. How
will this pregnancy be different from my earlier one?
There are several advantages to being older. You are more mature and
probably have more patience. Your financial situation may be better
than when you were younger. On the other hand, if you have problems
with chronic illness such as high blood pressure or diabetes, they can
worsen and affect both you and your baby.

Does this mean I shouldn't get pregnant now that I'm older?
No, but a pregnancy may be more difficult for you. This is a very individual
situation that you and your partner should discuss with your doctor.

I am 39 and hope to be pregnant soon. Will I need any special tests during pregnancy?
With increasing maternal age, tests to consider include ultrasound, amniocentesis, chorionic villus sampling, serum alpha-fetoprotein and diabetes testing.

What are some of the possible problems I might have if I am over 35 and get pregnant?
Risks are varied and include:

. an increased risk of a baby with Down's syndrome
. a higher risk of caesarean section
. problems with diabetes or high blood pressure
. a harder, longer labour

If you have other chronic medical problems, such as thyroid disease, or take medicines regularly, discuss your concerns with your doctor before getting pregnant.

My husband is older, and we've heard that his age can affect my pregnancy and our baby. Is this true?
Researchers believe this is true. It has been shown that chromosomal abnormalities occur more often in women over 35 and men over 40. Men over age 55 are twice as likely as younger men to father a child with Down's syndrome. However, the risk is small and chromosomal abnormalities can be detected if they do occur.

Nutrition before Pregnancy

I want to be pregnant soon. I love hamburgers, French fries and other junk foods. Will this be a problem when I get pregnant? I'll eat better then!
The best plan is to start eating nutritiously *before* you get pregnant. By the time many women know they're pregnant, they are 7 or 8 weeks into the pregnancy – or more! These early weeks of pregnancy are important in the development of your baby. Start eating properly before you become pregnant.

Can't I just start eating better when I find out I'm pregnant?
It is best for you and your developing baby if you develop good eating habits before you get pregnant. It is important to your health and the

development of your baby for you to eat nutritiously for the 12 months of pregnancy.

I plan to start watching my weight once I'm pregnant. Is there a problem with this plan?
Pregnancy is *not* the time to start a new diet or to try to lose weight. Dieting can cause temporary deficiencies in vitamins and minerals that are important to your developing baby. Ask your doctor about a good eating plan before getting pregnant, and make necessary changes before pregnancy.

Exercising before Pregnancy

I don't really like to work out. Is exercise that important?
Exercise is good for you, whether or not you are pregnant. Develop a good exercise programme before getting pregnant to help you feel better, control weight and increase stamina. Exercise can also help make labour and delivery easier.

How can I find and maintain a good exercise programme?
Find exercise you enjoy and can do in any type of weather. A great deal of information on various types of exercise programmes is available from your local hospital, your doctor and health clubs.

I love to exercise but have been warned about doing too much. How can I know if I am overdoing it?
Some general guidelines for exercise before and during pregnancy include:

• Before starting a new programme, consult your doctor about past medical problems and past pregnancy complications.
• Start exercising before you get pregnant.
• Exercise on a regular basis.
• Start gradually, and increase as you build strength.
• Wear comfortable clothing.
• Avoid contact sports or risky exercise, such as water skiing or riding.
• Allow plenty of time for warming up and cooling down.
• Check your pulse every 10 to 15 minutes during exercise.
• Don't let your pulse exceed 120 beats a minute.
• Once you're pregnant, be careful when changing positions.

- After the fourth month of pregnancy, don't lie flat on your back when exercising. This decreases blood flow to your baby.
- Stop exercising and consult your doctor if you have any bleeding, loss of fluid from the vagina, shortness of breath, dizziness, abdominal pain or other serious problems.

Substance Use

My friend just found out that she is 8 weeks pregnant. She uses cocaine once or twice a week but says she'll stop now that she's pregnant. Is this bad for the baby?
Any kind of substance abuse or drug use can be harmful during pregnancy. A woman should attempt to get these problems under control before stopping birth control or trying to conceive. A doctor can help a woman find assistance. It is extremely important to stop using cocaine before conceiving. Research has shown that damage to the baby can occur as early as 3 days after conception!

I've tried to stop smoking, but I don't know if I can. Can cigarette smoking harm a growing baby?
We know definitely that smoking affects pregnancy and development of the fetus. Low birth weight and a slow growth rate are problems in babies born to mothers who smoke. For your health and the health of your baby it's essential to stop smoking before you consider pregnancy.

My friend told me she stopped drinking before she got pregnant, but I don't drink very much. I don't have to stop, do I?
Although no harm has been shown from an intake of less than 12 units per week during preconception and pregnancy, some doctors believe it's best to abstain completely from alcohol during pregnancy. Every time you take a drink, your baby does too! It is also reasonable to stop using alcohol from the time you are preparing to conceive until after your baby is born.

There really aren't very many side effects from marijuana; I always feel relaxed when I smoke it. Is it bad for the baby?
It can be a dangerous drug during pregnancy. Marijuana crosses the placenta and enters the baby's system. We know it can cause attention deficits, impaired decision making and memory problems in childhood years if a fetus is exposed before birth.

Working before Pregnancy

At work I am exposed to an X-ray machine and chemicals every day. Will this be a problem when I am pregnant?
Get answers to these questions *before* you become pregnant. Many forms of exposure at the workplace, such as to X-rays and chemicals, could be harmful. If you wait to ask these questions until after you find out you're pregnant, you have already exposed your developing fetus to various dangers during some of the most important weeks of development.

My job requires me to stand for a 10-hour shift. I'm used to this, but will it be a problem when I'm pregnant?
Studies have shown that women who stand for a long time each day have smaller babies. If in the past you have had premature deliveries or an incompetent cervix (see also page 40), discuss the situation with your doctor.

Sexually Transmitted Diseases

In the last 2 years, I've had a chlamydia infection four times. Can this cause problems when I want to get pregnant in a few months?
Sexually transmitted diseases (STDs) can damage your uterus or fallopian tubes, making it more difficult to become pregnant. If you catch an STD while you're pregnant, it could affect your pregnancy.

How can I protect myself from STDs?
Having your partner use condoms is a good way to protect yourself against STDs, especially if you have more than one sexual partner.

What are some other sexually transmitted diseases?
Other STDs include gonorrhoea, genital herpes, genital warts (condylomata), syphilis and HIV (the virus that causes Aids). Before trying to get pregnant, use a condom if you have a problem with infections or are exposed to infections frequently, even if you use other forms of birth control. If you catch an infection, make sure it is cleared up before you try to become pregnant.

PART II

Your Pregnancy

CHAPTER 2

Your Health and Medical Concerns

I think I'm pregnant, but I'm not sure I know all the signs and symptoms of pregnancy. Can you tell me what to look for?
The first sign that you are pregnant will probably be a missed menstrual period. As your pregnancy progresses, you may experience:

- nausea, with or without vomiting
- fatigue
- breast changes and breast tenderness
- frequent urination

If am pregnant, is it true that my health can affect the health of my growing baby?
Yes. Good nutrition, proper exercise, sufficient rest and attention to how you take care of yourself all have an impact on your pregnancy. Your health care can also have an effect on your pregnancy and how well you tolerate being pregnant.

Someone said I should be in good health before I get pregnant. Why?
If you are in good health before you get pregnant, you'll feel more secure about your growing baby. You'll know that you've done your best to ensure a healthy baby.

When should I see my doctor?
It's best to see him or her before you become pregnant. Routine examinations will tell you that you are healthy and any problems are under control. If there are medical problems, they can be dealt with before your pregnancy begins.

What is Antenatal Care?

What is antenatal care, and why do I need it?

Antenatal means *before birth*, and *antenatal care* is the care you receive for your entire pregnancy. You need this special care to help you discover any problems before they become serious. Doctors and midwives are specially trained to deal with pregnancy and can answer your questions and deal with your concerns during this important time.

How does the care I receive affect my pregnancy?

You want to feel confident the care you receive is the best you can find. If you have confidence in your doctor, you will be able to relax and enjoy your pregnancy. It really is a special time in a woman's life, and an enjoyable one. You want to do everything possible to make it the best 9 months for your growing baby.

What can I expect on my first antenatal visit?

Your first antenatal visit may be your longest. You will be asked a lot of questions, and you will undergo a physical examination. Laboratory tests may be ordered.

What kind of questions will I be asked?

You will be asked for a complete medical history, including information about your periods, recent birth control methods and previous pregnancies. Tell your doctor or midwife about any miscarriages or abortions. Be sure to include information about hospital admissions or surgery you have had.

What other things will my doctor want to know?

Your doctor needs to know about any medicines you take or any medicines you are allergic to. Your family's past medical history may be important, such as the occurrence of diabetes or other chronic illnesses. Be sure to tell him or her about any chronic medical problems you have. If you have medical records, bring them with you.

I hate having a pelvic examination. Will I need one?

Yes, you probably will. A pelvic examination is important because it helps your doctor determine if your uterus is the appropriate size for your stage of pregnancy. A cervical smear will also be done, if it hasn't been done in the last year.

How often will I have to go to the doctor?
Most women go every four weeks for the first seven months, then every two weeks until the last month, then once a week. If problems arise, more frequent visits may be necessary.

What kind of laboratory tests will I need to have done?
Your doctor will probably order several tests during the first or second visit. These may include:

- a complete blood count
- urine analysis
- cervical smear (for cancer)
- cervical cultures, as indicated
- blood sugar test (for diabetes)
- rubella titres (for immunity against rubella)
- blood typing
- rhesus factor
- test for syphilis
- test for hepatitis antibodies
- alpha-fetoprotein test (for possible problems in the baby)

Choosing your Doctor

I have a friend who says I need to go to a special kind of doctor for antenatal care and delivery of my baby. Is this true?
You have many choices when it comes to choosing your doctor for your pregnancy. You can choose an obstetrician, a family practitioner or a certified midwife to oversee your antenatal care.

What is an obstetrician?
An *obstetrician* is a medical doctor who specialises in the care of pregnant women, including delivering babies. He or she has completed further training in obstetrics and gynaecology after medical school.

What is a family practitioner?
A *family practitioner* is sometimes called a *general practitioner* and often provides care for the entire family. Some family practitioners deliver babies and are very experienced at it. In some areas an obstetrician may not be available because the community is small or remote. In these cases, a family practitioner sometimes delivers babies. If problems arise, your family practitioner may refer you to an obstetrician for antenatal care.

What is a midwife?

A *midwife* is a trained professional who often cares for women who have low risk, uncomplicated pregnancies. These professionals are registered nurses who have sought additional professional training and qualification in midwifery. They are supervised by a doctor and call him or her if complications occur.

What is a perinatologist?

A *perinatologist* is an obstetrician who specialises in high risk pregnancies. Only about 10 per cent of all pregnant women need to see a perinatologist. If you have serious problems during pregnancy, you may be referred to a perinatologist. Or you may need to see one if you experienced problems with past pregnancies.

If I see a perinatologist, will my local hospital still deliver the baby?

This depends on the problem; it may still be possible for you to deliver at your local hospital. If you see a perinatologist, you may have to deliver your baby at a hospital other than the one you had chosen. Usually this is because of specialised facilities or the availability of specialised tests for you or your baby.

How can I find the best care giver for me?

If you have a hospital you like, you may not have to look any further. If you don't have one, call your doctor and ask for a referral. Ask friends who have recently had a baby about their hospital. Ask the opinion of a midwife. Sometimes another doctor, such as a paediatrician or physician, can refer you to an obstetrician. Ask your local librarian for publications that list maternity units in your area.

Who can I talk to about my fears and have answer my questions while I'm pregnant?

It's important to establish communication with your doctor or midwife so you can ask him or her *anything* about your condition. It's good to read articles and books as they help you prepare questions to ask your doctor. But *never* use any information you receive from other sources as a substitute for asking particular questions about your own pregnancy. Your doctor knows you, your history and what has occurred during this pregnancy. *Always* discuss your concerns with him or her!

I feel embarrassed asking some of the questions I have. They seem silly or stupid.

Don't be afraid to ask your doctor any question. He or she has probably already heard it, so don't be embarrassed. It's possible a situation is unwise or risky for you, so be sure to check even the smallest details. It's better to take time to get answers to all your questions than to wait until a problem develops.

Dealing with 'Morning Sickness'

I'm nauseated every morning but don't throw up. My friend had the same thing but had to go to the hospital for intravenous fluids. Is this 'morning sickness'?

An early symptom of pregnancy for many women is nausea, with or without vomiting; it is often called *morning sickness*. A condition called *hyperemesis gravidarum* results when a woman experiences a great deal of vomiting and the inability to eat foods or to drink fluids. If a woman has this problem, she may need to be treated in hospital with intravenous feeding and medicines for nausea.

I feel so nauseated in the morning that I can't eat anything. Does this last throughout pregnancy?

Nausea is typically at its worst during the beginning of pregnancy; most often it is bad in the morning and improves during the day. Morning sickness usually begins around week 6 and lasts until week 12 or 13, when it lessens and disappears.

What can I do about nausea?

Many things have been suggested to help you deal with the nausea and vomiting related to morning sickness. Try these suggestions, and use what works for you.

- Spread meals throughout the day so you eat several small snacks instead of one large meal.
- Eat a snack before you get up, such as crackers or rice cakes. Or ask your partner to make you some dry toast.
- Avoid heavy, fatty foods.
- Keep up your intake of fluids – they may be easier to handle than solids, and you want to avoid dehydration.
- Alternate wet foods with dry foods. Eat only dry foods at one meal,

then liquids at the next.
- Try ginger – it's a natural remedy for nausea. Grate it on vegetables and other foods.
- Suck on a cut, fresh lemon when you feel nauseated.
- Avoid things that trigger your nausea, such as odours, movement or noise.
- Get enough rest.
- Avoid getting sweaty or overheated, which can contribute to your nausea.

I have nausea and vomiting, but only at night. Is this the same thing as morning sickness?
Nausea and vomiting with pregnancy can occur at any time of the day or night; sometimes it lasts all day long. If often begins to lessen after a few weeks and usually disappears around the end of the first trimester.

My sister had to go into the hospital when she had morning sickness. Why?
If a woman gets dehydrated or loses a substantial amount of weight with morning sickness, she may have to be put in hospital where she can be fed intravenously. Usually it takes only a couple of days in hospital before the woman can resume eating solids. The main purpose of her going to hospital is to keep up her fluid intake and to give her the nourishment she needs through intravenous feedings.

One of my friends told me her dentist warned her to take care of her teeth if she had morning sickness. How were her teeth affected?
When nausea is accompanied by vomiting, the contents of the stomach that enter the mouth can cause a breakdown in tooth enamel. Brush your teeth after vomiting to remove any residue from the vomit.

How your Health affects your Growing Baby

How does my health affect my growing baby?
Your baby is totally dependent on you for all its needs. To make sure he or she gets the best possible start in life, it's important for you to eat well, get enough rest and stay as healthy as possible throughout your pregnancy.

I've heard that some infections and illnesses I have can affect the development of my baby. Is that true?

Yes. Some infections and illnesses you experience may affect your growing baby. That is why it is important to remind your doctor that you are pregnant when you call him or her about any medical problems. The chart on page 34 lists some of the more common ones, and the effects each illness can have on a developing fetus.

If I have a fever, especially a high one, can it hurt my baby?

Yes, it may. Your baby relies on you for its temperature control. A *prolonged* high fever, especially in the first trimester (first 13 weeks), can affect a developing fetus.

Is there anything I can do, which won't harm the baby, to bring down a high fever?

Drink lots of liquids, take paracetamol (Panadol) and dress appropriately to help you cool down. If your physician prescribes medicine for a cold, bladder infection or other illness, take it as prescribed.

I recently read that hepatitis is becoming more serious for pregnant woman. What do I need to be aware of?

Hepatitis is a viral infection of the liver and is one of the most serious infections that can occur during pregnancy. Your doctor will probably test you for hepatitis B at the beginning of your pregnancy.

How is hepatitis B transmitted?

Hepatitis B is spread from one person to another by the reuse of intravenous needles and by sexual contact and is the most common type of hepatitis. It can be transmitted to a developing fetus.

Are there other types of hepatitis?

Yes. They are named after the viruses that cause them. *Hepatitis A* is usually transmitted by person-to-person contact via poor sanitation or poor hygiene. It is responsible for about one-third of reported hepatitis cases.

Hepatitis C, also called *non-A, non-B hepatitis*, is responsible for about 10 per cent of hepatitis cases. You can become infected with this type of hepatitis through multiple blood transfusions or the use of intravenous drugs.

What are the symptoms of hepatitis?

Symptoms include flu-like symptoms, nausea and pain in the area of the liver or upper right abdomen. The person may appear yellow or jaundiced, and urine may be darker than normal.

How can hepatitis affect a developing baby?

Hepatitis is a viral infection that affects the liver. A developing baby that gets hepatitis is at serious risk of liver damage or stillbirth.

What can be done about this problem?

If a baby is born to a mother who tests positive for hepatitis at the beginning of pregnancy, it may be necessary to give the baby immune globulin against hepatitis after it is born. It is now recommended that all newborn babies receive hepatitis vaccine shortly after birth. Ask your doctor if the vaccine is available in your area.

I read that Group B streptococcus infection in a mother-to-be can cause lots of problems for her baby. What are some of them?

Group B streptococcus (GBS) rarely causes problems in adults but can cause life-threatening infections in the newborn, including pneumonia, meningitis, lung damage, kidney damage, loss of sight, hearing loss, cerebral palsy and developmental problems.

How could I get Group B streptococcus?

Group B streptococcus is often found in the mouth or lower-digestive, urinary or reproductive organs. In women, the bacteria are most often found in the vagina or rectum. You get an infection when your immunity or resistance is down. It is possible to 'carry' the bacteria in your system and not be sick or have any symptoms.

What are the symptoms of Group B streptococcus?

There may not be any symptoms. Sometimes a woman will have a vaginal discharge.

Can it be treated?

Yes, Group B streptococcus is treated with antibiotics.

Will I know I have Group B streptococcus?

We do not have an ideal screening test for vaginal Group B streptococcus. If you become high risk for developing this infection during labour, your doctor will test you at that time and give you antibiotics to help prevent transmission of the bacteria from you to your baby.

Why would I become high risk?
Your risk increases with premature labour, premature rupture of membranes or a previous Group B streptococcus infection.

Lyme disease is prevalent in our area. Is it dangerous for my baby if I get Lyme disease during my pregnancy?
Lyme disease is a rare infection caused by a spirochaete (bacterium) carried and transmitted to humans by ticks. We know the spirochaetes that cause Lyme disease do cross the placenta. Complications from this infection include preterm labour, fetal death or a rashlike illness in the newborn.

What are the symptoms of Lyme disease?
There are several stages of the disease. In most people, a skin lesion with a distinctive look, called a *bull's eye*, appears at the site of the bite. Flu-like symptoms appear, and after 4 to 6 weeks there may be signs of heart problems or neurological problems. Arthritis may be a problem later.

If I do get Lyme disease, how it is treated?
Treatment for Lyme disease includes long-term antibiotic therapy. Many medicines used to treat Lyme disease are safe for use during pregnancy.

How can I avoid exposure to Lyme disease?
Stay out of areas that are known to have ticks, such as heavily wooded areas. If you can't avoid them, wear long-sleeved shirts, trousers, socks and boots or closed shoes. Check your hair for ticks; they often attach themselves to the hair or the scalp.

What is lupus?
Lupus (systemic lupus erythematosus or *SLE)* is a disease of unknown cause that affects women more often than men (about 9 to 1). Women with lupus have a large number of antibodies in their bloodstream that are directed towards the women's own tissues. This can affect various parts of the body including the joints, skin, kidneys, muscles, lungs, brain and central nervous system.

Why is lupus a concern in pregnancy?
Lupus occurs most often in young or middle-aged women. Pregnant sufferers face a higher risk of miscarriage, premature delivery and complications around the time of delivery.

What are the symptoms of lupus?
The most common symptom is joint pain. Other symptoms include rashes or sores on the skin, fever, kidney problems and hypertension.

How is lupus treated?
The drugs of choice to treat lupus are steroids; the most commonly prescribed steroid is *prednisolone*. Many studies on the safety of prednisolone during pregnancy have found it to be safe.

I've heard a lot lately about toxic streptococcus A, the 'flesh-eating' bacteria. What is it?
Toxic streptococcus A can cause severe damage to anyone who suffers from it. It is a bacterial infection that usually starts in a cut on the skin, not as a sore throat. It spreads very quickly and can soon involve the entire body.

How might it get into my system?
The streptococcus A bacteria can get in through a very small scratch, scrape or cut in the skin. The skin turns red and becomes swollen, painful and infected very quickly.

What are the symptoms of toxic streptococcus A?
The symptoms include:

- fever above 102 °F (39 °C)
- an inflamed cut or scratch
- flu-like symptoms
- unusually cold extremities (feet, hands, legs and arms)

Is there anything I can do to prevent toxic streptococcus A?
Yes. Any time you cut or scratch yourself, clean the affected area with soap and water, alcohol or hydrogen peroxide. All are safe to use during pregnancy. After careful washing, apply an antibiotic cream or ointment (available over the counter) to the area. Use a light bandage if necessary. Keep the area clean, and reapply antibiotic ointment as needed. These same measures can and should be used with every member of your family.

I've been having some diarrhoea lately. Should I be concerned?

It's possible to have diarrhoea during pregnancy, and it can raise many concerns for you. If the diarrhoea doesn't go away in 24 hours, or if it keeps returning, contact your doctor. He or she may decide to have you take some medicine for the problem. Do not take any medicines for diarrhoea without first discussing it with your doctor.

Is there anything I can do myself if I have diarrhoea?

One of the best things you can do is increase your fluid intake. Drink a lot of water, juice and other clear fluids, such as broth. (Avoid apple juice, though, because it can act as a laxative.) You may feel better eating a bland diet, without solid foods, until you feel better.

Is it dangerous for my baby if I don't eat solids?

No, it isn't harmful for a few days provided you keep up your fluid intake. Solid foods may actually cause you more gastrointestinal distress. Avoid milk products while you have diarrhoea; they can make it worse.

My vet told me to be careful about contact with my cat. What does my cat have to do with my pregnancy?

If you have a cat, you may be exposed to *toxoplasma gondii*, a protozoan which causes *toxoplasmosis*. It is a disease that is spread by contact with infected cat faeces or by eating raw, infected meat. You can pick up protozoa from an infected cat's litter tray, from counters and other surfaces the cat walks on or from the cat itself when you pet it.

What problems can toxoplasmosis cause me or my baby?

Infection during pregnancy can lead to miscarriage or an infected infant at birth. Usually an infection in the mother has no symptoms.

How can I protect myself from toxoplasmosis?

A pregnant woman should avoid exposure to cat faeces. Get someone else to change the cat litter. Keep cats off work surfaces and other areas where you could pick up the protozoa. Wash your hands thoroughly after contact with your cat or contact with raw meat. Keep work surfaces clean, and cook meat thoroughly. Hygienic measures prevent transmission of the protozoa.

I've heard about cytomegalovirus. What is it?

Cytomegalovirus (CMV) is a member of the herpes virus family. It is transmitted in humans by contact with saliva or urine. Day-care centres are a common source of the infection. CMV can also be passed by sexual contact.

How can cytomegalovirus affect me?
Most infections do not cause any symptoms. When symptoms do occur, they include a fever, sore throat and joint pain.

How can cytomegalovirus affect my growing baby?
In an infant, CMV can cause low birth weight, microcephaly, calcification inside the skull, eye problems, mental retardation, motor retardation, jaundice, enlarged liver, enlarged spleen and anaemia.

I've heard about a pregnant woman getting rubella. What is it exactly?
Rubella, also called *German measles*, is a viral infection that causes few problems in the non-pregnant woman. It is more serious during pregnancy, especially in the first trimester.

What are the symptoms of rubella?
The most common symptom of rubella is a skin rash. You may also experience flu-like symptoms.

How can rubella affect my growing baby?
Rubella infection during pregnancy can increase the rate of miscarriage and cause malformations in the baby, especially heart defects.

I've been exposed to chicken pox. Can it hurt me or my baby?
If you have have chicken pox before, it shouldn't be a problem for either of you. If you haven't had chicken pox, this can be a problem. Exposure during the first trimester can result in birth defects, such as heart problems. Exposure close to delivery (within 1 week) can result in chicken pox in the baby.

How can chicken pox affect me?
Adults don't tolerate chicken pox as well as children. Contraction of the disease can result in serious symptoms, including painful lesions, high fever and severe flu-like symptoms.

I'm not sure if I've had chicken pox before. What can I do?
Avoid exposure to the disease, if you possibly can.

I have just read about varicella. What is it exactly?
Varicella (sometimes called *varicella-zoster*) is the member of the herpes virus family which causes chicken pox. Varicella may remain latent for years, only to be reactivated later as herpes zoster or shingles.

How can varicella affect me?
If you get shingles while you are pregnant, it can be a serious illness with severe pain and even breathing problems. Fortunately, it is rare.

What are the symptoms of varicella?
Pain is the main symptom of varicella (shingles); this may be accompanied by a rash or lesions.

How can varicella affect my growing baby?
It may cause birth defects. If you are exposed within two weeks of delivery the baby may catch the disease.

Environmental Poisons and Pollutants

I've heard that environmental poisons can be dangerous to a pregnant woman. What are they?
Environmental poisons and pollutants that can harm a developing fetus include lead, mercury, PCBs and pesticides. PCBs are polychlorinated biphenyls – byproducts of the plastics and electronics industries which were found to have contaminated some cooking oils and fish.

How can lead harm a developing baby?
Exposure to lead can cause an increase in the chance of miscarriage. Lead is readily transported across the placenta to the baby. Poisoning occurs as early as the 12th week of pregnancy.

How could I be exposed to lead?
Lead exposure may come from many sources, including some petrol, water pipes, solders, storage batteries, some construction materials, paints, dyes and wood preservatives. You may also be exposed in your workplace; find out if there is a risk.

How can mercury harm a developing baby?
Reports of mercury exposure have been linked to cerebral palsy and microcephaly.

Possible Antenatal Effects of Illness

Illness in Mother	*Possible Effect on Fetus*
Chicken pox	Heart problems
Cytomegalovirus	Microcephaly, brain damage, hearing loss
Group B streptococcus	Pneumonia, meningitis, cerebral palsy, damage to lungs or kidneys
Hepatitis	Liver damage, death
Lupus	Miscarriage, premature delivery
Lyme disease	Preterm labour, fetal death, rash in the newborn baby
Rubella (German measles)	Cataracts, deafness, heart lesions; can involve all organs
Syphilis	Skin defects, fetal death
Toxoplasmosis	Possible effects on all organs
Varicella	Possible effects on all organs

How could I be exposed to mercury?
Exposure usually occurs from contaminated fish. There was also a report of grain being contaminated with mercury.

How can PCBs (polychlorinated biphenyls) harm a developing baby?
PCBs are not single compounds but mixtures of several compounds. Most fish, birds and humans have small, measurable amounts of PCBs in their tissues. PCBs have been blamed in cases of miscarriage and fetal growth retardation.

How could I be exposed to PCBs?
We are exposed to PCBs through some of the foods we eat, such as fish.

How can pesticides harm a developing baby?
Pesticides have been held responsible for an increase in miscarriage and fetal growth retardation.

How could I be exposed to pesticides?
Pesticides include a large number of agents used to control unwanted plants and animals. Human exposure is common because of the extensive use of pesticides. Those of most concern include DDT, chlordane, heptachlor and lindane (Quellada).

How can I protect myself against these agents?
The safest course is to avoid exposure, whether by oral ingestion or through the air you breathe. Thoroughly wash all fruits and vegetables before eating. It may not be possible to eliminate all contact. If you know you will be exposed to certain chemicals, be sure to wash your hands thoroughly afterwards.

Discomforts of Pregnancy

I've had a lot of problems with heartburn during my pregnancy. What causes it?
Discomfort from heartburn is one of the most common complaints during pregnancy. It may begin early in pregnancy, although it generally becomes more severe as pregnancy progresses. Heartburn is caused by reflux (regurgitation) of stomach contents into the oesophagus.

I don't usually have heartburn when I'm not pregnant. Why does it occur so much during pregnancy?

It occurs more frequently during pregnancy because of two factors – decreased gastrointestinal function or movement (motility) and compression of the stomach by the uterus as it grows larger and moves up into the abdomen.

Is there anything I can do about heartburn?

Antacids may provide considerable relief. Follow the directions relating to pregnancy on the package or ask your doctor. Don't overdo it and take too much in an effort to find relief. You can use some antacids, such as Gaviscon, Gelusil, Milk of Magnesia and Maalox, without much concern. Avoid sodium bicarbonate as it may cause you to retain water. In addition to use of antacids, the following tips may provide some relief:

- Eat smaller, more frequent meals.
- Avoid eating before bedtime.
- When lying down, elevate your head and shoulders.

Can the foods I eat affect my heartburn?

Some foods can affect your heartburn. Try to find foods (and amounts) that don't give you heartburn. Eliminate foods that cause you problems. Add foods that benefit you and your growing baby.

What's the difference between heartburn and indigestion?

Indigestion refers to the inability to digest food or difficulty digesting food. *Heartburn* is a burning discomfort related to the lower end of the oesophagus and is felt behind the lower part of the sternum (breastbone).

If I have indigestion, is there anything I can do about it?

Eat foods that agree with you; avoid spicy foods. Eat small meals frequently. If you need them, take antacids after meals, but don't over-do this.

I never had haemorrhoids before my pregnancy, but now I do. Why?

Haemorrhoids are very common during pregnancy. They are caused by the increased, congested blood flow in the pelvis because of the increased weight and size of the uterus.

What exactly are haemorrhoids?
They are dilated blood vessels around the area of the anus or up inside the anus. They can itch, bleed and be painful.

What can I do about haemorrhoids?
Eat adequate amounts of fibre and drink lots of fluid. Salt baths help, and suppository medicines, available without a prescription, can provide relief. You may need stool softeners. If haemorrhoids become a major problem for you, consult your doctor.

I have headaches but don't want to take any medicine I don't have to during pregnancy. What can I do about them?
It's a good idea to try to deal with your problem without medicines. There are several things you can try that are medicine-free.

- Use deep breathing exercises and relaxation techniques to help you relax.
- Close your eyes and rest in a quiet place.
- Eat regularly. Avoid foods or substances, such as caffeine, that might cause a headache.
- Apply an ice pack to the back of your head.
- Get enough sleep.

If my headaches won't go away using these techniques, is there any medicine I can take?
Paracetamol (Panadol) is recommended for headaches. You can take the regular or extra strength version. If this doesn't help, call your doctor.

I suffer from migraine headaches. What can I do about them during pregnancy?
Migraine headaches during pregnancy are not unusual. Try the techniques described above. If they don't help, discuss the problem with your doctor. Do *not* take any medicine for a migraine headache without first discussing it with your doctor.

I have problems with allergies. Will they cause me problems during pregnancy?
Your allergies may change with your pregnancy. Sometimes they become more pronounced, sometimes less.

What can I do for my allergies while I'm pregnant?
Drink plenty of fluid, especially during hot weather. If there are foods you're sensitive to, be more careful what you eat. This also applies to other things you might be sensitive to, such as animals or cigarette smoke.

Can I take regular allergy medicines while I'm pregnant?
Ask your doctor or pharmacist before taking any medicine; don't assume it's all right, even if it is available over the counter. It's safer and easier to ask beforehand rather than taking a chance with any medicine.

My nose has been stuffed up ever since I got pregnant. Is this normal?
Some women complain of nasal stuffiness or nosebleeds during pregnancy. We believe these occur because of circulation changes caused by hormonal changes in pregnancy. These can make the mucous membranes of the nose and nasal passages swell and bleed more easily.

What can I do about my stuffed-up-nose?
Do *not* use decongestants or nasal sprays to relieve stuffiness. Many are combinations of several drugs that should not be used during pregnancy. Try a humidifier to relieve stuffiness. Increase your fluid intake, and use a gentle lubricant, such as petroleum jelly. Discuss it with your doctor if these remedies don't provide relief.

Special Concerns of Pregnancy

My mother told me to discuss my rhesus factor with my doctor. Why?
You may be rhesus negative, which requires some additional attention during pregnancy and after your baby is born.

What does it mean to be rhesus negative?
Your blood type, such as O, A, B, AB, contains a factor that determines if it is positive or negative. In the past, rhesus negative women who carried a rhesus positive baby faced complicated pregnancies that could result in a very sick child. Today, most of these problems can be prevented. If you are rhesus negative, you need to know it.

Why is being rhesus negative a problem?
If you are rhesus negative and your baby is rhesus positive, if you have had a blood transfusion or received blood products of some kind, you could become rhesus-sensitised or isoimmunised. This could affect the baby.

What does it mean to be 'isoimmunised'?
If you are *isoimmunised*, you have antibodies that circulate inside your system. They won't harm you, but they can attack the blood of a rhesus positive fetus. Antibodies from you can cross the placenta and attack your baby's blood. This can make your baby anaemic while it is still inside the uterus and can be very serious.

How does a woman become sensitised?
A rhesus negative woman becomes sensitised when rhesus positive blood gets into her bloodstream. This can happen with a blood transfusion with rhesus positive blood, the birth of a rhesus positive baby, a miscarriage or an ectopic pregnancy.

What can I do about this problem?
Many problems can be prevented with the use of anti-D immunoglobulin, which is rhesus-immune globulin. If you are rhesus negative and pregnant, an injection of anti-D immunoglobulin is given at 28 weeks of pregnancy to prevent sensitisation before delivery.

When is it used after the birth?
Within 72 hours after delivery, you will be given a second injection of anti-D immunoglobulin if your baby is rhesus positive.

Not all babies are rhesus positive, are they?
No. Some women who are rhesus negative carry a child who is also rhesus negative. In this case, no anti-D immunoglobulin injection is given after delivery.

Are there other situations in which anti-D immunoglobulin is used?
Yes. if you have an ectopic pregnancy and are rhesus negative, you should receive anti-D immunoglobulin. This also applies to miscarriages and abortions. If you are rhesus negative and have amniocentesis, you will also receive anti-D immunoglobulin.

A woman I met at my doctor's surgery told me she had an 'incompetent cervix' with her last pregnancy. What is that?
An *incompetent cervix* is a condition in which a woman has painless dilatation (stretching) of the cervix that occurs prematurely. In most cases it is unnoticed by the woman. Membranes may rupture without any warning, and this usually results in premature delivery of the baby.

How will I know if this is happening to me?
The problem is not usually diagnosed until *after* one or more deliveries of a premature baby without any pain before delivery. If it's your first pregnancy, there is no way for you to know if you have an incompetent cervix.

What causes an incompetent cervix?
Some researchers believe it occurs because of previous trauma to the cervix, such as D and C (dilatation and curettage) for an abortion or after a miscarriage. It may also occur if surgery has been performed on the cervix.

If this problem occurs, is there any treatment for it?
Treatment is usually surgical. A weak cervix can be reinforced by sewing the cervix shut. When the woman goes into labour, the suture is opened and the baby can be born normally.

At my last appointment my doctor said my blood pressure was up. Should I be concerned?
It is normal for your blood pressure to change a little during pregnancy. It often decreases a little during the second trimester of pregnancy and increases towards the end of pregnancy.

What can I do about high blood pressure if it becomes a problem?
Resting in bed on your side can help. If your blood pressure is still too high, drugs may be necessary to lower it.

I'm dizzy a lot. Should I worry?
Feeling dizzy while you're pregnant is a fairly common symptom. Anaemia can cause dizziness any time during pregnancy and can be diagnosed with a blood count (see also page 43). Another cause of dizziness is *hypotension* (low blood pressure). Hypotension in pregnancy usually occurs during the second trimester.

What causes hypotension in pregnancy?

There are two causes of hypotension during pregnancy. It can be caused by the enlarging uterus putting pressure on large blood vessels, such as your aorta and vena cava. This is called *supine hypotension* and may happen when you lie down. It can be alleviated or prevented by not sleeping or lying on your back.

The second cause of hypotension is rising rapidly from a sitting, kneeling or squatting position; this is called *postural hypotension*. When you rise rapidly, gravity causes blood to leave your brain, which may result in a drop in blood pressure. This is avoided by rising slowly from a sitting or lying position.

Can problems with my blood sugar cause dizziness?

Yes. Pregnancy affects your blood sugar; either high blood sugar (*hyperglycaemia*) or low blood sugar (*hypoglycaemia*) can make you feel dizzy or faint. Many doctors routinely test pregnant women for problems with blood sugar.

If I have a problem with blood sugar, what can I do?

The problem can be avoided or improved by eating a balanced diet, not skipping meals and not going a long time without eating. If it is more serious, you may need to see a dietician. If blood tests show diabetes, see a specialist.

My sister had pregnancy-induced hypertension. What is it?

Pregnancy-induced hypertension is high blood pressure that occurs only during pregnancy. It will disappear after the baby is born. It develops in about 3 per cent of women under age 40, and in 10 per cent of women over 40.

What can be done about pregnancy-induced hypertension?

It is treated with bed rest, drinking lots of fluid and avoiding salt and foods containing large amounts of sodium. Drugs to lower blood pressure may be prescribed. For further information, see the discussion of *pre-eclampsia* in Chapter 15.

What is the difference between a urinary tract infection (UTI) and a bladder infection?

UTI refers to an infection anywhere in the urinary tract, including the bladder, the urethra, the ureters and the kidneys. A *bladder infection* refers to an infection in the bladder only. The terms are often used interchangeably.

Why do I get more bladder infections now that I'm pregnant?
This happens because of changes in your urinary tract. The uterus sits directly on top of the bladder and on the tubes leading from the kidneys to the bladder, called *ureters*. As the uterus grows, its increased weight can block the drainage of urine from the bladder and cause an increase in bladder infections. From 5 to 10 per cent of pregnant women will experience bladder infections.

How does my doctor check for bladder infections?
Usually your doctor will do a urine analysis and culture on your first visit. He or she may also check your urine for infections on subsequent visits.

What are the symptoms of a bladder infection?
Symptoms of a bladder infection include:

• frequent urination
• burning urination
• feeling as though you need to urinate and nothing will come out
• blood in your urine (with severe infection)

I've heard about a more serious urinary tract infection called pyelonephritis. What is it?
Pyelonephritis is an infection of the urinary tract that also involves the kidneys. It occurs in 1–2 per cent of all pregnant women.

What are the symptoms of pyelonephritis?
Symptoms of pyelonephritis include:

• frequent urination
• burning urination
• feeling as though you need to urinate and nothing will come out
• high fever
• chills
• back pain
• blood in the urine

How is pyelonephritis treated?
Pyelonephritis may require hospital admission and treatment with intravenous antibiotics.

How often do kidney stones occur during pregnancy?
Kidney stones, also called *urinary calculi*, occur about once in every 1,500 pregnancies.

What are the symptoms of a kidney stone?
Symptoms usually include severe pain in the back and blood in the urine.

How is a kidney stone diagnosed?
In pregnancy, ultrasound is generally used to diagnose a kidney stone.

How is a kidney stone treated?
A kidney stone in pregnancy can usually be treated with pain medication and by drinking lots of fluid or receiving intravenous fluids.

I've read about a procedure called lithotripsy that is used to treat kidney stones. What is it?
Lithotripsy uses electronically generated shock waves to crush a kidney stone in the bladder or urethra. It is not normally used during pregnancy.

Anaemia during Pregnancy

My doctor says I have anaemia now that I'm pregnant. What is it?
Anaemia is a common medical problem in many pregnant women. The number of red blood cells in your blood is low; the quantity of these cells is inadequate to provide the oxygen needed by your body.

Why does anaemia occur so often in pregnancy?
Your blood volume increases by about 35 per cent during pregnancy. Blood is made up of fluid and cells. The fluid usually increases faster than the cells. This may result in a drop in your haemoglobin and the volume, amount or percentage of red cells in the blood. The drop can result in anaemia.

Why is it important to treat anaemia during pregnancy?
If you suffer from anaemia, you won't feel well during pregnancy, and you'll tire more easily. You may also experience dizziness. If you're anaemic when you go into labour, you're also at a higher risk of needing a blood transfusion when your baby is born. Pregnancy

anaemia can cause an increased risk of preterm delivery, growth retardation in the baby and low birth weight. Your doctor will tell you if you are anaemic and prescribe a course of treatment for you.

What is the most common type of anaemia during pregnancy?

The most common type of anaemia during pregnancy is *iron deficiency anaemia*. While you are pregnant, your baby uses some of your iron stores. With iron deficiency anaemia, your body does not make enough red blood cells to keep up with the increased demand.

What causes iron deficiency anaemia?

Several factors can cause this condition, including:

• bleeding during pregnancy
• multiple fetuses (twins, triplets)
• recent surgery on your stomach or small bowel
• frequent antacid use
• poor dietary habits

Is iron-deficiency anaemia easy to control?

Yes, it usually is. Iron is contained in most antenatal vitamins. If you can't take antenatal vitamins, you may be given iron supplementation. Eating certain foods, such as liver or spinach, also helps increase the amount of iron you take in.

I've heard about sickle cell anaemia. What is it?

Sickle cell anaemia occurs when a person's bone marrow makes abnormal red blood cells. It occurs most often in black people or those of mixed-black descent.

How do I know if I have sickle cell anaemia?

Your doctor can perform a blood test to see if you have this disease.

Doesn't sickle cell anaemia also cause pain?

Yes, it can cause pain in the abdomen or limbs of the mother-to-be if she has a *sickle crisis*. This can happen at any time in her lifetime, not just during pregnancy.

Are there any other problems with sickle cell anaemia?

In addition to a painful sickle crisis, the mother-to-be can suffer from more frequent infections and even congestive heart failure. Risks to the fetus include a higher incidence of miscarriage and stillbirth.

What is thalassaemia?

It is a type of anaemia that occurs most often in people of Mediterranean descent. The body doesn't produce enough globulin that makes up the red blood cells, so anaemia results. If you have a family history of thalassaemia, discuss it with your doctor.

Your Pre-existing Medical Problems

I have diabetes. How does it affect my pregnancy?

Diabetes was once a very serious medical problem during pregnancy. It continues to be an important complication, but today a woman can go safely through a pregnancy if she has proper medical care, watches her diet and follows her doctor's instructions. Using a glucometer to measure your blood sugar is a good practice.

What are the symptoms of diabetes?

The symptoms of diabetes include:

- an increase in urination
- blurred vision
- weight loss
- dizziness
- increased hunger

Why is diabetes serious in pregnancy?

Diabetes can cause several medical problems including kidney problems, eye problems, blood problems and heart problems, such as hardening of the arteries. Any of these can be very serious for you and your baby. If diabetes is not treated, you will expose your baby to a high concentration of sugar. This is called *hyperglycaemia* and is not healthy for the baby.

Why is diabetes a problem for the baby?

If you have uncontrolled diabetes, you face a significant increase in the risk of miscarriage and of major fetal development abnormalities if the pregnancy continues. The most common fetal problems are heart problems, genito-urinary problems and gastrointestinal problems.

How is diabetes diagnosed?

Diabetes is diagnosed with a blood test called a fasting blood sugar or with a glucose tolerance test.

If there is sugar in my urine, does it mean I have diabetes?

No, not necessarily. It is common for normal, pregnant, non-diabetic women to have a small amount of sugar in their urine, called *glucosuria*. This occurs because of changes in your sugar levels and the way sugar is handled in the kidneys during pregnancy.

I have epilepsy, and I have just found out I'm pregnant. I'm very excited about the pregnancy, but I'm really concerned about the medicine I take. What should I do?

Call your doctor *immediately*; tell him or her you are pregnant and you have epilepsy. Most medicines to control seizures can be taken during pregnancy. However, some medicines are safer than others.

What medicines are all right to use?

During pregnancy, phenobarbitone is often used to control seizures. Phenytoin (Epanutin) is not recommended for controlling seizures because it can cause birth defects in a baby. Discuss this important issue with your doctor as soon as possible.

I suffer from asthma. Can I have a safe pregnancy even if I have problems with my asthma?

Most women who have asthma can have a safe pregnancy. If you have severe asthma attacks before pregnancy, you may have them during pregnancy. Usually the medicines you take before pregnancy can be taken while you are pregnant. Discuss this with your doctor.

Besides taking my medicine, is there anything else I can do for my asthma during pregnancy?

We've found that many women feel better and have fewer problems with their asthma if they increase their fluid intake during pregnancy. Try it – you should increase your fluid intake during pregnancy anyway.

A pregnant woman I know has just found out she has cancer. Isn't this uncommon?

You're right; cancer during pregnancy is *not* common. Many cancers in women occur after menopause, which lowers the overall likelihood of cancer in pregnancy. However, cancer does occur during pregnancy, but rarely.

I hate to think about cancer during pregnancy. Should I be concerned about it?

I agree with you – it's not a very pleasant subject to think about or discuss, and most women do not need to be concerned about it. However, it's better to be aware that these problems can occur than not to know anything about them.

What is the most common type of cancer discovered during pregnancy?

The most common cancer found is breast cancer. Gynaecological cancers, leukaemia, lymphoma, melanoma and bone tumours are also found.

Is there any reason these cancers might appear during pregnancy?

Researchers believe there are two main reasons why cancers could appear during pregnancy.

- Some cancers arise from tissues or organs that are influenced by the increase in hormone levels caused by pregnancy.
- Increased blood flow and changes in the lymphatic system may contribute to the spread of cancer to other parts of the body.

I've heard it's harder to find breast cancer during pregnancy. Why?

Changes in the breasts, including breast tenderness, increased size and even lumpiness, may make it harder to discover this type of cancer. Of all women who have breast cancer, about 2 per cent are pregnant when it is diagnosed.

How is breast cancer treated during pregnancy?

Treatment varies. It could be surgery, chemotherapy, radiation or a combination of treatments.

If a woman has breast cancer, can she breast feed?

Most doctors recommend a woman not to breast feed if she has breast cancer.

Are treatments for cancer during pregnancy dangerous?

Cancer treatments can cause problems, including miscarriage, fetal death, fetal malformations and fetal growth retardation. The pregnant woman may also experience side effects from the treatment.

I've been having chemotherapy for 6 months and have just found out I'm 8 weeks pregnant. What should I do?
It's very important to talk to your doctor immediately! What you will do depends on the medicines you are taking.

Other Medical Concerns

I get awful leg cramps at night. What can I do about them?
Leg cramps, especially at night, can be very bothersome. The following may help you deal with the problem.

- Wear support tights during the day.
- Take warm baths.
- Have your partner massage your legs at the end of the day or whenever you feel like it.
- Wear comfortable clothing.
- Take paracetamol (Panadol) for pain.
- Rest on your side.
- Use a heat pad for up to 15 minutes when you experience pain.

Can my activities affect my leg cramps?
Yes, they can. Avoid standing for long periods of time. Rest and lie on your side as often as possible. Make sure clothing is not restrictive.

Before pregnancy, I often visited a chiropractor for back pain. Can I go to a chiropractor if I have back pain during pregnancy?
Low back pain is common during pregnancy – nearly half of all pregnant women suffer from it. If you have severe problems that you believe might be helped by chiropractic manipulation, discuss it with your regular doctor *before* you do anything! Whatever you do, avoid X-rays of your pelvic and lower back area.

I'm almost 36 and about 7 weeks pregnant. Is there anything I should worry about because of my age?
Today, more couples are waiting to start their families, so you're not alone. There are increased risks for the older mother-to-be and her baby, but it's still very likely that you and your baby will be all right. The risks include Down's syndrome, high blood pressure, caesarean section delivery, multiple births, pre-eclampsia, placental abruption, bleeding and other complications.

I'm 35 and pregnant with my third child. I'm a lot more tired than I remember being before. What's wrong with me?

Putting it simply, it's harder to be pregnant when you're 35 than it is when you're 25. It doesn't necessarily mean anything is wrong.

I'm over 35. What are my chances of having a baby with Down's syndrome?

As you get older, the risk of delivering a baby with Down's syndrome increases. Look at the following statistics:

- at age 25 the risk is 1 in 1,300 births
- at 30 it is 1 in 965 births
- at 35 it is 1 in 365 births
- at 40 it is 1 in 109 births
- at 45 it is 1 in 32 births
- at 49 it is 1 in 12 births

But let's look at in a more positive light. If you're 45, you have a 97 per cent chance of *not* having a baby born with Down's syndrome. If you're 49, you have a 92 per cent chance of delivering a child without Down's syndrome. It is still important that over the age of 35 you have a blood test to confirm that the risk is very low. Over the age of 40 it is essential that you have an amniocentesis or similar test to check that your baby does not have Down's syndrome.

CHAPTER 3

Tests on You and your Growing Baby

I am really anxious to be pregnant. How far along must I be for a pregnancy test to be positive?

Pregnancy tests have become increasingly sensitive and can be positive (pregnant) even before you miss a menstrual period. Most tests will be positive 7 to 10 days after you conceive; this includes blood, urine and home pregnancy tests. Most doctors recommend you wait until you miss your period before having a test. This will save you both money and emotional energy.

I did a home pregnancy test last night, and it was positive. How soon should I see my doctor?

Once you know you're pregnant, call and make an appointment. Most doctors will want to see you within a few weeks unless you are having problems and need to be seen right away. Good antenatal care is an important part of having a healthy baby. Don't wait for weeks or months to see your doctor; starting early is important for your health and the health of your baby.

My friend had a pregnancy test called a quantitative HCG test because she was having problems; the result was a number. What kind of test is it?

A *quantitative HCG (human chorionic gonadotrophin) test* is a blood test done in the first trimester when there is concern about miscarriage or ectopic pregnancy. The test measures the hormone HCG, which is made early in pregnancy and increases rapidly. Two or more tests done a few days apart are more useful than one test because it is the *change* in the amount of the hormone that is significant. An ultrasound scan is also often done when a quantitative HCG test is ordered.

My doctor said I'm going to have to have a lot of tests done when I go in next time. What kind of tests will I need?
Your doctor will probably order several tests during the first or second visit. These may include:

• complete blood count
• urine analysis and culture
• test for syphilis
• cervical cultures, as indicated
• rubella titres (for immunity against rubella)
• blood type
• rhesus factor
• test for hepatitis B
• alpha-fetoprotein test
• ultrasound
• cervical smear

See the chart on page 71 for a description of some common tests done during pregnancy.

Why do I need to have all these tests?
The results of these tests give your doctor the information he or she needs to provide the best care for you. For example, if testing shows you have never had rubella (German measles) or rubella vaccine, you will know you need to avoid exposure and receive the vaccine before your next pregnancy. Rubella can be responsible for miscarriage or fetal malformations if a woman contracts the disease during pregnancy.

I'm 28 weeks pregnant, and my doctor says I need some more tests. Why?
Many doctors repeat some tests or perform new tests at this time. For example, the 28th week of pregnancy is the best time to discover any abnormalities in glucose tolerance. It is at this point in your pregnancy that anti-D immunoglobulin is given to a rhesus negative woman to protect her from becoming sensitised.

I'm pregnant for the first time and want everything to be all right. Do I need genetic counselling?
Probably not. Individuals who need genetic counselling are usually those who have had a malformed baby, those with a family history of inherited diseases and women who have had recurrent miscarriages (usually three or more).

What happens when a couple goes for a genetic counselling?
You and your partner will participate in this counselling together. Detailed questions will be asked about your medical history, other pregnancies, medicines you take and the medical history of your family and your partner's family. If it is necessary to do chromosome tests, blood samples will be taken from both of you.

Ultrasound

All my friends have had ultrasound scans during pregnancy. Will I have one?
Many doctors routinely perform ultrasound scans on their patients, but not every doctor does them with every patient. Some doctors perform them only when there is a problem or a definite reason for doing one.

I'm confused about ultrasound and sonograms. What's the difference?
Ultrasound, sonogram and *sonography* refer to the same test. Ultrasound is a valuable medical tool, especially in pregnancy.

Ultrasound technician or doctor

Screen where picture is seen

Transducer

Ultrasound examination is a useful aid that your doctor may order for you.

This ultrasound picture shows a baby's profile inside the uterus.

What exactly is an ultrasound scan?

An *ultrasound scan* is a test that gives a 2-dimensional picture of the developing embryo or fetus. It involves the use of high frequency sound waves made by applying an alternating current to a transducer. This transducer is placed on the abdomen or in the vagina. Sound waves projected from the transducer travel through the abdomen or vagina, bounce off tissues and bounce back to the transducer. The reflected sound waves are translated into a rough picture.

Is an ultrasound test safe?

Yes, it is. Most medical researchers agree that ultrasound examinations pose no threat to you or your baby. The possibility of ultrasound having effects has been studied many times without evidence that the test causes any problems.

Why do doctors do ultrasound scans?

There are three main reasons that your doctor will arrange for you to have an ultrasound scan:

• to help confirm or determine your due date
• to determine whether there is more than one baby (twins, triplets or more)
• to see if major physical characteristics of the fetus are normal

Will I automatically have an ultrasound scan?

No. Whether you have an ultrasound scan during your pregnancy depends on several factors. These factors include:

- problems during pregnancy, such as bleeding
- previous problem pregnancies
- your doctor

Most doctors like to do at least one ultrasound scan during a pregnancy, but not all agree on this. If your pregnancy is 'high risk', you may have several ultrasound scans.

Are there other reasons for doing an ultrasound scan?

Some other reasons for doing an ultrasound scan are:

- identifying an early pregnancy
- showing the size and growth of the embryo or fetus
- measuring the fetal head, abdomen or thighbone to determine the duration of pregnancy
- identifying some fetuses with Down's syndrome
- identifying fetal abnormalities, such as hydrocephalus
- measuring the amount of amniotic fluid
- identifying the location, the size and the maturity of the placenta
- identifying abnormalities of the placenta
- detecting an intra-uterine contraceptive device
- differentiating between miscarriage, ectopic pregnancy and normal pregnancy
- helping to find a safe location to perform an amniocentesis

How early in pregnancy can I have an ultrasound scan?

That depends on your doctor. If you're having problems, he or she may want you to have an ultrasound scan fairly early in pregnancy.

Can an ultrasound scan help determine when I'm due?

Yes. Measurements can be taken of the baby with ultrasound. Your doctor can compare these measurements with charts that have averages to help approximate your due date.

Will I be able to find out if I am having a boy or girl when I have my ultrasound scan?

If you are 18 weeks or more when you have an ultrasound scan, you *may* be able to determine the sex of your baby, but don't count on it.

Ultrasound scan of male scrotum and penis at 33 weeks.

It isn't always possible to tell the sex if the baby has its legs crossed or is in a breech presentation.

Even if your doctor makes a prediction as to the sex of your baby, keep in mind that ultrasound is a test, and tests can sometimes be wrong. Most doctors recommend you not to start buying for one sex or the other based on an ultrasound scan. If you do buy anything, save the receipts!

I've heard that sometimes the ultrasound instrument is put in the vagina. Is that dangerous; could it make me bleed or miscarry?
This type of ultrasound scan is called *vaginal ultrasound* and can be very helpful in evaluating problems early in pregnancy, such as possible miscarriage or an ectopic pregnancy. The instrument (probe or transducer) is put just inside the opening of the vagina, so it does not touch the cervix and will not cause bleeding or miscarriage. This type of ultrasound scan can sometimes give better information earlier in pregnancy than an abdominal scan.

I'm supposed to have an ultrasound scan next week, and they told me to drink 2 pints (1 litre) of water before I come and not to empty my bladder. Why?
Your bladder is in front of your uterus. When your bladder is full, your uterus rises out of the pelvis and can be seen more easily. When your bladder is empty, your uterus is further down in your pelvis, and it's harder to see it. The full bladder acts as a window from the outside of

your abdomen into your uterus. With a vaginal ultrasound scan, your bladder doesn't have to be full.

Where are most ultrasound scans done?

There are three locations where ultrasounds are usually done.

- Some doctors have an ultrasound machine in their clinic and have ultrasound training.
- Some doctors prefer to have you go to the hospital ultrasound department to have the scan done and read by a radiologist.
- In certain high risk situations, your doctor may send you to an ultrasound specialist at another hospital.

Each situation must be considered individually; ask your doctor about where your ultrasound will be done.

My friend has a videotape of her ultrasound scan. Can I get one of mine?

Ask about it when your ultrasound scan is scheduled. Not all ultrasound machines are capable of making a video recording. Ask ahead of time to find out if you need to bring a videotape.

Can I get pictures from my ultrasound scan?

Most ultrasounds include black-and-white photos. Baby pictures before you have a baby!

I'm having an ultrasound scan next week. Can my partner come with me?

Yes. This is something your partner will probably want to see, so arrange to have the scan when he can come. You may want to have others, such as your mother or older children, come when possible. Ask about this when your scan is scheduled.

Amniocentesis

I heard some women talking about amniocentesis. Is this test for everyone?

No, *amniocentesis* does not need to be performed on every pregnant woman. It is usually performed on women who:

- will deliver after their 37th birthday

- have had a blood test showing an increased risk of Down's syndrome
- have had a previous baby with a birth defect
- have a family history of birth defects
- have a birth defect themselves
- have a partner with a birth defect

When is the test done?
Amniocentesis is usually performed for antenatal evaluation between 16 and 18 weeks of pregnancy.

How is amniocentesis performed?
Ultrasound is used to locate a pocket of fluid where the fetus and placenta are not in the way. Skin over the abdomen is cleaned and numbed with a local anaesthetic. A needle is passed through the abdomen into the uterus, and fluid is withdrawn from the amniotic cavity with a syringe.

How much fluid is withdrawn?
Only about 1fl oz (30ml) of amniotic fluid is needed to perform the tests.

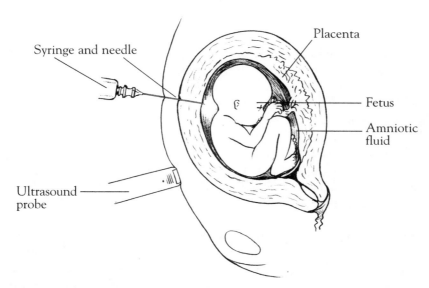

Amniocentesis is usually performed between the 16th and 18th weeks of pregnancy.

What do they do with the amniotic fluid?
Fetal cells that float in the amniotic fluid can be grown in cultures. These cells can then be used to confirm that your baby is healthy or to identify fetal abnormalities.

How many abnormalities can amniocentesis identify?
We know there are over 400 abnormalities a child can be born with. Amniocentesis can identify about 10 per cent of them, or 40 problems.

What kind of abnormalities can be found with amniocentesis?
The problems a doctor can identify include the following:

• chromosomal problems, particularly Down's syndrome
• skeletal diseases, such as osteogenesis imperfecta
• fetal infections, such as herpes or rubella
• central nervous system diseases, such as anencephaly
• blood diseases, such as erythroblastosis fetalis
• chemical problems or deficiencies, such as cystinuria or maple syrup urine disease

Can't amniocentesis also determine the baby's sex?
Yes it can. However, the test is not used for this purpose, except in cases in which the sex of the baby could predict a problem, such as haemophilia.

What are the risks of this test?
Risks are relatively small, but there could be trauma to the fetus, placenta or umbilical cord, infection, miscarriage or premature labour. Fetal loss from complications is estimated to be about 0.5–3 per cent. Discuss it with your doctor before you have the test.

Who performs amniocentesis?
The test should be performed *only* by someone who has experience doing it, such as a doctor at a hospital. Your own doctor will be able to give you more information about this.

I keep hearing about Down's syndrome. What is it exactly?
Down's syndrome is a condition caused by a defect in the baby's chromosomes. The baby will be mentally retarded and may have a somewhat dwarfed appearance, with a sloping forehead, short, broad hands, a flat nose and low-set ears. He or she may also have heart

problems, gastrointestinal defects or leukaemia. Down's syndrome can be diagnosed during pregnancy by amniocentesis.

Is there a way to diagnose Down's syndrome without doing amniocentesis?
Yes. Studies are now being done with other tests that can diagnose Down's syndrome. These tests include alpha-fetoprotein, chorionic villus sampling and ultrasound (in some cases).

The Alpha-fetoprotein Test

A friend told me about a blood test she had that can detect problems with the baby. What is it?
You probably mean the *alpha-fetoprotein (AFP)* test. It is a blood test done on *you* to determine an abnormality in your *baby*! Measurement of the amount of alpha-fetoprotein in your blood can help your doctor predict problems.

Is the AFP test done on all pregnant women?
At present it is not performed on all pregnant women. If the test is not offered to you, discuss it with your doctor.

When is the test done?
It is usually performed between 16 and 20 weeks of pregnancy, and test results must be correlated with the mother-to-be's age and weight and the gestational age of the fetus. If AFP detects some problem, additional, more definitive testing is usually ordered.

What kind of abnormalities can AFP detect?
The test is designed to detect babies with:

. neural tube defects
. severe kidney disease
. severe liver disease .
. oesophageal or intestinal blockage
. Down's syndrome
. urinary obstruction
. osteogenesis imperfecta (fragility of the baby's bones)

I've heard that if I have an alpha-fetoprotein test, there is a chance that it will be abnormal, even if there are no problems. Is this true?
Yes, this is true. The problem with the test is that it is not specific enough. For example, if 1,000 women are tested, some 40 tests will come back abnormal. Of those 40 tests, only one or two actually have a problem. So if you have an AFP test and the result is abnormal, don't panic. Another AFP test will be done to correlate results, and an ultrasound scan will be performed.

What is a neural tube defect?
A *neural tube defect* is an abnormality in the bone surrounding the spinal cord, in the brain stem or in the brain itself. One of the most common neural tube defects is *spina bifida* – an absence of vertebral arches, which allows the spinal membrane to protrude. Another abnormality is *anencephaly*; the brain develops only a rudimentary brain stem and only traces of basal ganglia, in the lower part of the brain.

Chorionic Villus Sampling

I've heard about a test called chorionic villus sampling. What is it?
Chorionic villus sampling (CVS) is a test that is done to detect genetic abnormalities. Sampling is done early in pregnancy, usually between the 9th and 11th weeks.

How is the test done?
A small piece of tissue is removed from the placental area with an instrument placed through the cervix or with a needle inserted through the abdomen.

Are there risks in having CVS done?
There is a small risk of miscarriage with this procedure. The test should be performed *only* by someone who is experienced in doing it.

Why is this test ordered?
The advantage of CVS is that it can provide an earlier diagnosis of a problem, if one exists. The test can determine various fetal problems, such as Down's syndrome, Tay-Sachs disease and cystic fibrosis. Some women choose to have this test because they want results in good time to make decisions about the pregnancy.

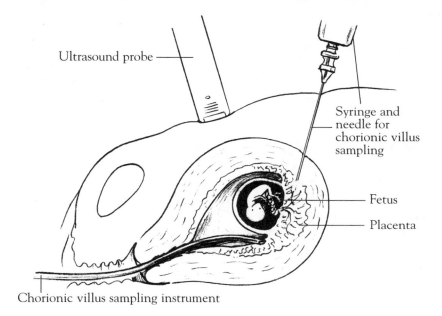

Ultrasound probe

Syringe and needle for chorionic villus sampling

Fetus

Placenta

Chorionic villus sampling instrument

Chorionic villus sampling can be done earlier in pregnancy than other tests and is a valuable tool for your doctor.

Is CVS better than amniocentesis?
CVS does offer an advantage over amniocentesis because it can be done much earlier in pregnancy. Results are available in about a week. If the woman decides to terminate the pregnancy after learning the results of the test, the procedure can be performed earlier in pregnancy and may carry fewer risks. On the other hand, the risk of disturbing a normal pregnancy is slighting higher with CVS than with amniocentesis.

Should I have this test done?
Each woman's pregnancy is different. This test should be discussed with your doctor. He or she will be able to determine if your particular case requires it.

Fetoscopy

What's the test that uses some kind of '-scope' to look at the baby?
You are probably referring to *fetoscopy*. It is performed on the fetus and
placenta while both are still inside your uterus. It provides a view of
the baby and placenta.

What is fetoscopy used for?
The doctor can actually see the baby through the fetoscope, and some
abnormalities and problems can be detected. This very specialised test
is not performed very often.

How is the procedure done?
A small incision is made in the mother's abdomen, and the instrument
is placed through the abdomen. The doctor uses the fetoscope to
examine the fetus and placenta.

Should I have fetoscopy?
If you doctor suggests fetoscopy to you, discuss it with him or her. This
test is *not* done very often, but is used when it is necessary to look
directly at the fetus or placenta.

Are there risks to fetoscopy?
Risk of miscarriage is 3–4 per cent with this procedure. The test should
be done *only* by someone experienced in this technique.

Other Tests for the Mother-to-be

**My friend told me about a special stethoscope that my doctor will use
to let me hear my baby's heart beat. What is it?**
You're probably referring to a special listening machine called a
doppler. It is not actually a stethoscope. It magnifies the sound of the
baby's heartbeat enough so you can hear it.

When will I be able to hear the baby's heartbeat?
Around the 12 week visit this will be possible. If your doctor doesn't
offer it to you, ask about it.

I'm concerned about having tests that use radiation during my pregnancy. Can they hurt my baby?

Avoid exposure to X-rays during pregnancy, unless it is an emergency. There is no known safe amount of radiation for a developing fetus. Dangers to the baby include a very small increase in the risk of mutations and of cancer later in life.

I have to go to the dentist next week. Should I let them X-ray my teeth?

If possible, avoid dental X-rays while you are pregnant. However, if you *must* have a dental X-ray, be sure your abdomen and pelvis are completely shielded by a lead apron.

What should I do if I break my leg and need an X-ray while I'm pregnant?

There *are* medical reasons for X-rays, but the need for the X-ray must be weighed against the very small risk to your pregnancy. If you have an injury to your foot or hand, it is fairly easy to shield the uterus with a lead apron while the area is X-rayed. However, if your injury is in your back or any place near the pelvic area, the risks increase. When you are pregnant, discuss any X-ray with your doctor before it is taken.

Are there any other reasons to do an X-ray during pregnancy?

Some problems, other than broken bones, may occur that require X-rays. Pneumonia and appendicitis are two possibilities. Again, discuss the situation with your doctor.

What about CT scans – are they the same as X-rays?

Computerised tomographic scans, also called *CT scans* and *CAT scans*, are a form of very specialised X-ray. The technique involves the use of X-ray with computer analysis. Many researchers believe the amount of radiation received from a CT scan is much lower than a regular X-ray. However, it is probably wise to avoid even this amount of exposure, if possible.

When is the fetus most susceptible to the harmful effects of radiation from X-rays?

Risk to a fetus appears to be greatest between 8 and 15 weeks of pregnancy (between the fetal ages of 6 and 13 weeks). Some believe the only safe amount of radiation exposure for a fetus is no exposure.

I've heard about a test called MRI. Is it the same as an X-ray?

No. *Magnetic resonance imaging*, also called *MRI*, is a diagnostic tool widely used today. So far no harmful effects in pregnancy have been reported from its use, but pregnant women are advised to avoid an MRI during the first trimester of pregnancy for the safety of the fetus.

I'm going for my first visit, and the surgery told me that the doctor will want to do a cervical smear. What is a cervical smear?

A cervical smear involves the removal of some cells from your vagina or cervix. It is done to look for abnormal cells, called *precancerous*, *dysplastic* or *cancerous* cells, in the cervix.

Why does the doctor do a cervical smear at this time?

If you have had a normal cervical smear in the last few months, you won't need it. If it has been a year or more since you had the test, you should have a cervical smear. The goal of a cervical smear is to find problems early so that they can be more easily dealt with.

I saw my doctor a week ago, and the surgery has just called to tell me my cervical smear wasn't normal. Will I need a biopsy?

It depends on how serious the problem might be. Usually a biopsy is not done while you're pregnant. Your doctor will probably wait until after your pregnancy for further testing. Instead of removing tissue for a biopsy, he or she may do a *colposcopy* (a very careful look at the cervix) during pregnancy. An abnormal cervical smear during pregnancy is a very individual situation and must be handled carefully.

What is home uterine monitoring?

With home uterine monitoring, contractions of a pregnant woman's uterus are monitored in her home. This type of testing or monitoring is sometimes used when the doctor believes there could be a problem with premature labour. If necessary, labour would be stopped to prevent delivery of a premature baby.

How does home uterine monitoring work?

A recording of uterine contractions is transmitted from the woman's home, via telephone, to a centre where contractions can be evaluated. With the use of a personal computer, your doctor may be able to view the recordings at his or her own home or office.

Who needs home uterine monitoring?
Conditions that may require home uterine monitoring include:

- previous preterm delivery
- infections in the mother-to-be
- premature rupture of membranes
- pregnancy-induced hypertension
- multiple fetuses, such as twins or triplets

My doctor wants me to have a cardiotocogram (CTG). What is that?
A *cardiotocogram* is a non-invasive procedure done in the doctor's surgery, in the labour room or in the delivery room. While you are lying down, a fetal monitor is attached to your abdomen. Every time you feel the baby move, you push a button to make a mark on the monitor paper. At the same time, the fetal monitor records the baby's heart beat on the same paper.

What will a cardiotocogram show?
The information gained from a cardiotocogram gives reassurance that your baby is doing all right.

A cardiotocogram and a contraction stress test are done to evaluate the fetus.

External fetal monitoring, with membranes intact (bag of waters has not broken).

If my cardiotocogram isn't all right, what happens next?
Additional tests may be done, including a *biophysical profile* or a *contraction stress test*.

I'm close to delivery, and my doctor said I will have a pelvic examination the next time I come to the surgery. Why now, when I haven't had one for so long?
A pelvic examination is needed late in pregnancy because it tells us a lot of things, including:

- presentation of the baby – whether the baby is head first or breech
- dilatation of the cervix – how much the cervix has opened (if at all)
- effacement – how much the cervix has thinned
- shape and size of your birth canal or pelvic bones
- station – how low the baby is in your birth canal

After my pelvic examination, my doctor said I was '2 and 50 per cent'. Why did she tell me this?
This information is important for two reasons. First, it tells you your cervix is open 2cm (about 1in) and thinned out 50 per cent or halfway. (This is not an indication of when your baby will be born.) Secondly, this information is helpful if you go to the hospital thinking you're in labour. At the hospital, you'll be checked again. Knowing what you were

at your last pelvic examination can help determine if you are in labour.

My doctor did a pelvic examination today and told me my cervix was not dilated and had not thinned out. Does that mean I have a lot longer to go?
No. The pelvic examination tells you where you were at *that* time. Labour may begin at any time.

When my doctor does a pelvic examination, does that tell him when I will go into labour?
No. At this point in your pregnancy, labour might start at any time, no matter what the condition of your cervix.

My doctor was mentioning fetal monitoring during labour and delivery. What is it?
In many hospitals, a baby's heart beat is monitored throughout labour to detect any problems early so they can be resolved.

What kind of monitoring do they do?
There are two types of fetal monitoring during labour – *external fetal monitoring* and *internal fetal monitoring* with a scalp electrode (see the illustrations on the page opposite and below.

Internal fetal monitoring during labour with a scalp electrode. Membranes (bag of waters) have ruptured.

What is external fetal monitoring?

A belt with a receiver is strapped to your abdomen, and it records the baby's heart beat. This type of monitoring can be done before your membranes rupture.

What is internal fetal monitoring?

Internal fetal monitoring is a more precise method of monitoring the baby. An electrode is placed on the fetal scalp to give a more exact reading of the fetal heart rate than that from external monitoring.

Tests for your Developing Baby

My doctor mentioned doing a biophysical profile on my baby. What is it?

It is a comprehensive test that examines the fetus while it is still in your uterus. It helps determine the baby's health.

Why is a biophysical profile done?

The test is useful in evaluating a fetus with intra-uterine growth retardation, when the mother-to-be is diabetic, with a pregnancy in which the baby doesn't move very much, in high risk pregnancies and in overdue pregnancies.

What does a biophysical profile measure?

It measures and records:

- fetal breathing movements
- body movements
- fetal tone (tightening or contractability of muscles)
- reactive fetal heart rate (increase in heart rate when baby moves)
- amount of amniotic fluid

How is the test performed?

The test is done with various instruments. Ultrasound, external monitors and observation are used to make the different measurements.

How is the test scored?

Each area is given a score of 0, 1 or 2. A total is obtained by adding all five scores together. The higher the score, the better the baby's condition. A low score may indicate problems in the fetus.

If a baby has a low score, what can be done?
The situation will be evaluated – the baby may need to be delivered immediately. If the score is reassuring, the test may be repeated at intervals. It may be necessary to repeat the test the following day. Your doctor will evaluate the scores, your health and the entire pregnancy before any decisions are made.

I've heard about a contraction stress test for the baby. What is that?
A *contraction stress test (CST)*, also called a *stress test*, is another test that is used to evaluated the well-being of the baby.

How is a contraction stress test done?
A monitor is placed on the woman's abdomen to record the fetal heart rate. Sometimes nipple stimulation is used to make the woman's uterus contract, or an intravenous fluid infusion is started and oxytocin is given in small amounts to make the uterus contract. Results indicate how well a baby will tolerate contractions and labour.

What can a contraction stress test indicate?
If the baby doesn't respond well to the contractions, it can be a sign of fetal distress.

When is a contraction stress test done?
If a woman has had problem pregnancies in the past or experiences medical problems during her present pregnancy, her doctor may have her tested in the last few weeks of pregnancy. This is done when the cardiotocogram is not reassuring.

I recently read about fetal blood sampling during labour. What is this test?
It is another way of evaluating how well a baby is tolerating the stress of labour.

How is fetal blood sampling during labour done?
The membranes must have ruptured, and the cervix must be dilated at least 2cm (about 1in). An instrument is placed inside the mother to make a small nick in the baby's scalp. The baby's blood is collected in a small tube, and its pH (acidity) is checked.

What can the doctor learn from fetal blood sampling?
The pH level can help determine whether the baby is having trouble during labour and is under stress. The test helps the physician decide whether labour can continue or if a caesarean section needs to be done.

I've heard about some test they can do to see if a baby is ready to be born; it has something to do with the baby's lungs. Why is it done?
You are probably referring to two tests that are done to evaluate the maturity of fetal lungs. When a baby is born prematurely, a common problem is immaturity of the lungs, which can lead to development of respiratory distress syndrome in the baby. The lungs are not completely mature, and the baby cannot breathe on its own without assistance.

Why is it important for the baby's lungs to be mature?
The last fetal system that matures is the respiratory system. If your doctor knows the baby's lungs are mature, it aids him or her in making a decision about early delivery.

What tests can be done to check fetal lung maturity?
One called an *L/S ratio* measures the ratio of lecithin to sphingomyelin. Results give the doctor an index of the maturity of the baby's lungs. The other is the *phosphatidyl glycerol (PG) test*, which gives a positive or negative result. Both tests are performed by amniocentesis. If the result shows phosphatidyl glycerol is present, there is greater assurance that the baby will not develop respiratory distress syndrome.

If the baby's lungs have not developed enough, what can be done?
The first course of action is to avoid premature delivery of the baby, if possible. If this cannot be done, a drug called dexamethasone may be injected into the mother to help mature the fetal lungs. Tests are done immediately after birth to determine if the baby has surfactant in its lungs. *Surfactant* is a chemical essential for respiration immediately after birth. If it is not present, the baby's doctor may introduce surfactant directly into the lungs of the newborn, preventing respiratory distress syndrome. The baby will not have to be put on a respirator – it can breathe on its own!

Some Common Tests at a Glance		
Test	How It's Done	What You and your Doctor Can Learn
Ultrasound	Sound waves produce picture of uterus, placenta and fetus on the screen	Age of fetal growth, fetal position, heart rate, movement, number of fetuses, some birth defects, fetal sex (sometimes)
Alpha-fetoprotein	Blood sample drawn from mother	May indicate neural tube defect (spina bifida) or risk of Down's syndrome
Amniocentesis	Sample of amniotic fluid drawn by needle from uterus	Early in pregnancy indicates chromosomal problems (Down's syndrome), neural tube defects (spina bifida), genetic disorders (cystic fibrosis), sex of fetus; late in pregnancy indicates whether baby's lungs are developed.
Chorionic villus sampling	Sample of placental tissue drawn from placenta through abdomen or vagina	Used to determine many inherited diseases, such as Down's syndrome, and some biochemical diseases, such as Tay-Sachs disease, and other fetal conditions such as cystic fibrosis
Cardiotocogram	Fetal activity is monitored by mother-to-be and fetal monitor	Used to show fetal well-being or to look for fetal stress
Biophysical profile	Variety of tests, including ultrasound monitoring and observation	Used to show fetal well-being or to look for fetal stress

CHAPTER 4

Medicines and Treatments for You

When should I discuss with my doctor the different medicines that I must take for the medical conditions I have?
Ideally, you will have had this discussion with your doctor *before* you got pregnant. If you were unable to do this, tell your doctor on your first visit about all medicines (prescription and over-the-counter) you take on a regular basis. Doses may need to be adjusted, or you may have to stop taking a particular substance.

Can't I just stop taking the medicine I take before I visit the doctor? I'm not that sick.
Never stop taking any medicine that you take for a chronic problem without first consulting your doctor. Some medicine cannot and should not be stopped during pregnancy. Consult your doctor before making any decisions about medicines.

I've read that some of the medicines I take can affect my growing baby. What are they and what are the effects?
The substances you ingest affect the developing baby in many ways. See the chart on page 75, which lists some of these substances and their effects.

Vitamin Use during Pregnancy
(Also see the discussion of vitamin use in Chapter 5)

How important is it for me to take antenatal vitamins?
It's very important to take your antenatal vitamins for your entire pregnancy. Sometimes late in pregnancy a woman stops taking them –

she gets tired of taking them or she decides they aren't necessary. The vitamins and iron in antenatal vitamins are essential to the well-being of your baby, so be sure you take your antenatal vitamins until your baby is born.

I usually take a lot of vitamins, but my doctor advised me to take only an antenatal vitamin during pregnancy. Why?

Too much of a good thing can be harmful. Some vitamins accumulate in your body's tissues when taken in megadoses and can have an adverse effect on you and your baby. Researchers believe that megadoses of vitamin A can cause birth defects when taken during pregnancy. In addition, we believe vitamins D, E and K in megadoses can also be harmful. Follow your doctor's advice, and eat nutritious, well-balanced meals to get the vitamins and minerals you and your baby need.

My friend is pregnant, and she's taking folic acid in addition to her antenatal vitamins. Is that something I need to do?

Some women do not need to take extra folic acid during pregnancy. (Folic acid is found naturally in green leafy vegetables.) However, a deficiency in folate (the term used interchangeably with folic acid) at the start of pregnancy has been linked with a small proportion of fetal abnormalities and it is now recommended that all women planning a pregnancy should take 0.4mg a day, continued through the first 12 weeks of pregnancy, to prevent this. Some doctors recommend continuing this throughout pregnancy to prevent a type of anaemia called megaloblastic anaemia. Additional folate may be necessary in situations in which requirements are unusually high, such as twins, triplets, epilepsy treated with drugs, Crohn's disease or alcoholism. If you take a antenatal vitamin preparation, check that it supplies 0.4mg of folic acid a day.

I've read that if a woman has a baby with spina bifida, she needs extra folic acid in subsequent pregnancies. Is that true?

Studies indicate a woman who has had a baby with a neural tube defect, such as spina bifida, can reduce her chances of having another baby with the same problems if extra folic acid is taken before pregnancy and through early pregnancy.

Prescription Medicines during Pregnancy

Why should I discuss the prescription medicines I take with my doctor?
This is a very important aspect of your antenatal care. Discuss *all* medicines (prescription and over-the-counter) you take on a regular basis on your first visit to your doctor. You may need to have your dose adjusted, you may have to stop taking a particular substance or certain conditions may require additional medicine.

I take thyroid medicine. Is it necessary during pregnancy?
Yes, it is very important to continue taking your thyroid medicine throughout your pregnancy. Be sure your doctor knows what you take.

Why is thyroid medicine important in pregnancy?
Thyroid hormone is made in the thyroid gland, which is found in your neck over the area of your windpipe. This hormone affects your entire body and is important in your metabolism. Thyroid hormone is also important in your ability to get pregnant.

Can medicines for thyroid problems be taken safely during pregnancy?
Thyroxine (medicine for low thyroid or hypothyroid) can be taken. Propylthiouracil (high thyroid or hyperthyroid medicine) passes to the baby; you will probably be given the lowest amount possible during your pregnancy.

I have lupus, and I take pills every day. Can this affect my pregnancy?
The medicines used to treat lupus are steroids; the primary steroid given is prednisolone. Many studies have been done on the safety of prednisolone during pregnancy, and it has been found to be safe.

Before pregnancy, I was taking fluoxetine (Prozac) for depression. Can I continue taking it?
There is little information about this drug's use or safety. Discuss taking fluoxetine with your doctor as soon as you discover you are pregnant.

Possible Effects of Some Medicines on the Fetus

Medicine	Possible Effects
Androgens (male hormones)	Ambiguous genital development (depends on dose given and time when given)
Anti-coagulants (warfarin)	Bone and hand abnormalities intra-uterine growth retardation, central nervous system abnormalities, eye abnormalities
Anti-thyroid drugs (propylthiouracil, iodine, methimazole)	Hypothyroidism, fetal goitre
Chemotherapeutic drugs (methotrexate, aminopterin)	Increased risk of miscarriage and fetal abnormalities
Isotretinoin (Roaccutane)	Increased miscarriage rate, nervous-system defects, facial defects, cleft palate
Lithium	Congenital heart disease
Phenytoin (Epanutin)	Growth retardation, mental retardation, microcephaly
Stilboestrol	Abnormalities of female reproductive organs, female and male infertility
Streptomycin	Hearing loss, cranial nerve damage
Tetracycline	Hypoplasia of tooth enamel, discoloration of first teeth
Thalidomide	Severe limb defects
Trimethadione	Cleft lip, cleft palate, growth retardation, miscarriage
Valproic acid	Neural tube defects

Chart modified from ACOG Technical Bulletin #84, Teratology, 2/85, American College of Obstetricians and Gynecologists

I asked my doctor for a prescription for isotretinoin (Roaccutane) to treat my acne, but she told me she couldn't prescribe it because I'm pregnant. Why?

Isotretinoin is a common treatment for acne. However, it must not be taken by any woman who is pregnant! There is a higher frequency of miscarriage and malformation of the fetus if a woman takes Roaccutane during the first trimester of pregnancy.

I use tretinoin (Retin-A, Rettinova) for my skin. Should I discontinue using it now that I'm pregnant?

This treatment is too new for us to know whether it is safe to use during pregnancy. We do know that any type of medicine you use can get into your bloodstream and could be passed to your baby. It's best to avoid tretinoin during pregnancy because we do not at this time know its effects on the fetus.

I often take tetracycline for a skin problem, but my brother warned me it can harm my baby. How?

None of the tetracyclines, a family of antibiotics, should be taken during pregnancy. They can cause discolouration of your baby's first teeth. For that reason, tetracyclines should also *not* be prescribed for any child under age 8.

I occasionally use a steroid cream for a skin condition I have. Can I use it during pregnancy?

It's best to discuss this with your doctor. There may be another preparation you can use that is considered safer during pregnancy.

Non-prescription or Over-the-counter medicines

Is it all right for a pregnant woman to take medicines that don't require a prescription?

Over-the-counter medicines (OTCs) should be taken with care during pregnancy. Ask your doctor about any medicine *before* you take it, whether it is prescription or non-prescription. Many OTCs contain aspirin, caffeine or phenacetin – all should be avoided during pregnancy. Limit your use of cough syrups, which may contain as much as 25 per cent alcohol. Be careful with medicines containing ibuprofen, such as Brufen, Fenbid, Nurofen and Codafen. Avoid new medicines, such as naproxen (Naprasyn, Nycopren, Synflex, Napratec) until we know more about them and their safety in pregnancy. Read package labels and ask your doctor or pharmacist before taking anything.

What are some safe non-prescription medicines?
Medicines that are safe include paracetamol (Panadol) and some antacids such as Gaviscon, Gelusil, Maalox and Milk of Magnesia.

Is it all right for me to take aspirin during my pregnancy?
Almost any medicine you take when you are pregnant passes to your baby or has some effect on your pregnancy. Even with a non-prescription medicine such as aspirin, it's best to consult your doctor before taking it.

Won't my doctor or the nurses get mad if I call them about every medicine I'm thinking of taking?
No. They would rather answer a question about which medicine to use before you take something than worry about its effect on your baby after you have taken it.

Can Birth Control Methods affect Pregnancy?

I have just found out I'm pregnant, and I'm taking birth control pills. What should I do?
Stop taking the pills, and notify your doctor. Any method of contraception can fail; the chance of failure with birth control pills is less than 1 to 3 per cent. There may be a small increase in problems for the fetus if you take birth control pills while you're pregnant. It is not cause for great alarm, but discuss it with your doctor.

I have a coil (an intra-uterine contraceptive device) and have just found out I'm pregnant. What should I do?
Notify your doctor immediately. You will need to discuss with him or her whether the coil should be removed. Most doctors will attempt to remove the coil if it comes out easily. The risk of miscarriage is higher if your coil is left in place. The risk of ectopic pregnancy is also higher if you get pregnant with a coil in place.

My partner uses condoms and spermicides, and I have just found out I'm pregnant. Will the fact that we have been using spermicides hurt our baby?
Spermicides have not been shown to be harmful to a developing fetus.

Immunisations and Vaccinations in Pregnancy

I've heard I should be careful about immunisations and vaccinations during pregnancy. Why?
Some immunisations may harm the developing fetus and should not be received by a pregnant woman. The risk of exposure to various diseases is an important consideration, however, and not all vaccines can cause harm to the fetus. That's why it is very important to discuss the matter with your doctor.

If I do need an immunisation, what will my doctor do?
Once your doctor determines you have been exposed to a disease, or exposure is possible, he or she will weigh the risk of the disease against the potentially harmful effects of the immunisation. As I've already stated, some vaccines *are not harmful* to a fetus and may be used without problems.

Are there some vaccines that I should never receive if I know I'm pregnant.
Yes. Live virus vaccines should *never* be given to a pregnant woman. Live virus vaccines include those for measles, mumps and rubella, poliomyelitis and yellow fever. You should receive primary vaccine against polio *only* if your risk of exposure is high, as it would be if you were travelling to a high risk area.

What types of vaccines are given to people?
The categories of vaccines are:

- live virus (mumps vaccine)
- inactivated virus (influenza, hepatitis B)
- inactivated bacterial (cholera, plague)
- toxoids (tetanus, diphtheria)
- specific immune globulins (rabies)
- standard immune globulins (hepatitis A)

Are any vaccines regarded as safe for a pregnant woman?
The only vaccines generally regarded as completely safe during pregnancy are tetanus and diphtheria. Others may be safe, but we are unsure about them at present, so avoid them.

How can I find out if I should receive a vaccine?
If you are pregnant, ask your doctor. If you don't think you are pregnant, it would still be wise to have a pregnancy test and to be using reliable contraception before receiving a vaccine.

There are so many different kinds of medicine. How can I remember which are safe to take?
You don't have to remember them all. Ask your doctor about those that pertain to your own special case. Much of the information in this chapter probably won't apply to you, but it's good information to have at hand. The important thing is to call your doctor about any non-prescription medication before you take it. And remember to read labels!

CHAPTER 5

Nutrition, Exercise and Weight Management

I've heard that during pregnancy I'm 'eating for two'. I this true?
What the old adage 'a pregnant woman is eating for two' actually means is that you must be concerned about nutrition for yourself and for your growing baby. However, many women take this to mean they can eat *twice as much*, which is incorrect! Be smart about your food choices – you must eat wisely for both of you.

Can't I eat all I want during pregnancy?
Only a very few lucky women can eat all they want at any time. Some women have the false idea they can eat all they want during pregnancy. Don't fall into this trap. You don't want to gain more weight than your doctor recommends during your pregnancy – it can make you uncomfortable and it will be harder to lose the extra pounds after your baby is born.

Why is it important for me to eat well during pregnancy?
In one study, it was shown that 95 per cent of the women who had good to excellent diets had babies in good to excellent health. Of women who ate poor diets (lots of junk food), only 8 per cent had babies in good to excellent health. One of your main goals in pregnancy is to have the healthiest baby you can. Your nutrition during pregnancy has a great impact on your baby's health.

Do I need to increase the number of calories I consume now that I'm pregnant?
Yes. Most experts say a normal weight pregnant woman needs to increase her calorie intake by 300–800 calories a day. These extra calories are important for tissue growth in you and your baby. Your

baby is using the energy from your calories to create and store protein, fat and carbohydrates and to provide energy for its own body processes. Expect to gain some weight during your pregnancy – it's natural and normal.

What foods should I eat every day?

A variety of foods should be included to supply you with the nutrients you need. You'll want to eat dairy products, protein foods, fruits and vegetables, and breads and cereals.

I don't think I eat very many foods with protein in them. Why should I eat foods containing protein?

During pregnancy you need protein for growth and development of the fetus, placenta, uterus and breasts. The recommended amount of protein in pregnancy is 6–7oz (168–196g) a day.

How many grams of carbohydrate should I eat daily during pregnancy?

There is no recommended dietary allowance for carbohydrate intake during pregnancy. Most doctors believe carbohydrates should make up about 60 per cent of the total number of calories in your diet. If you are eating 2,000 calories a day, you would consume about 1,200 calories as carbohydrate.

Do I need to worry about getting enough fat in my diet during pregnancy?

There is rarely concern about inadequate fat intake; usually fat intake is excessive. There is no recommended daily amount for fat intake during pregnancy.

I read that everyone has to have fat in their diet. I shouldn't avoid all fats, should I?

That's a good point. No, you shouldn't avoid all fats, but you should include them only in small amounts. Measure how much you use of each, and use them sparingly!

I'm confused about what I should eat every day. Can you recommend a healthy eating plan?

It's a good idea to eat a variety of foods throughout your pregnancy. Below is a list of daily portions from six food groups.

- Dairy products: 4–5 portions a day
- Protein sources: 3–4 portions a day
- Vegetables: at least 4 portions a day
- Fruits: 2–4 portions a day
- Breads, cereal, pasta and rice: 6–11 portions a day
- Fats/flavourings: 3–5 portions a day

What kinds of foods are dairy products, and how much should I eat of each?
Try these foods in the following amounts:

- 6oz (170g) cottage cheese
- 2oz (60g) processed cheese
- 1¹/₂oz (40g) natural cheese (such as Cheddar)
- 1oz (30g) hard cheese (such as Parmesan or Romano)
- 8oz (240ml) pudding or custard
- glass of milk 8oz (240ml)
- 8oz (240ml) yogurt

To keep the fat content low, choose skimmed milk, low fat yogurt and low fat cheese instead of whole milk and ice cream.

What kinds of foods are good sources of protein, and how much should I eat of each?
Try these foods in the following amounts:

- 2 tbsp (30g) peanut butter
- 4oz (120g) cooked dried beans
- 2–3oz (60–90g) cooked meat
- 1 egg

Aim for a total of 6–7oz (170–200g) daily. Poultry, fish, lean cuts of red meat, dried beans, eggs, nuts and seeds are all good sources of protein.

What kinds of foods are in the vegetable group, and how much should I eat of each?
Try these foods in the following amounts:

- 6oz (170ml) vegetable juice
- 4oz (120g) broccoli, carrots or other vegetable, cooked or raw
- 1 medium baked potato
- 8oz (240g) raw, leafy vegetables (salad greens)

Eating a variety of vegetables gives you a good nutritional balance. Eat at least one vegetable a day that is high in folic acid, such as green leafy vegetables.

What kinds of foods are in the fruit group, and how much should I eat of each?
Try these foods in the following amounts:

- 4oz (120g) tinned or cooked fruit
- 6oz (170g) grapes
- 4oz (120ml) fruit juice
- 1 medium banana, orange or apple
- 2oz (60g) dried fruit

Include one or two servings of a fruit rich in vitamin C, such as orange juice or orange slices. Fresh fruits are also a good source of fibre which is important during your pregnancy if you suffer from constipation.

What kinds of foods are in the bread-pasta-cereal-rice group, and how much should I eat of each?
Try these foods in the following amounts:

- 4oz (120g) cooked pasta, cereal or rice
- 1oz (30g) ready-to-eat cereal
- 1 slice bread
- 1 medium bread roll

What kinds of foods are in the fat/flavourings group, and how much should I eat of each?
Try these foods in the following amounts:

- 1 tablespoonful (15ml) sugar or honey
- 1 tablespoonful (15ml) olive oil or other type of oil
- 1 pat of margarine or butter
- 1 tablespoonful (15ml) jam
- 1 tablespoonful (15ml) prepared salad dressing

Be a little more careful in your use of these foods because they can be troublesome when you are trying to control your weight.

I have a hard time avoiding foods that are high in sugar and fat. What can I do?
Foods such as biscuits, chocolate, sweets and ice cream have a lot of calories. Fill up instead on foods that are high in fibre and low in sugar

and fat. Choose fruits and vegetables, pulses and whole-grain biscuits and breads.

I really love protein foods that have a lot of fat, like bacon and cheeses. What can I substitute for them?
Choose foods that are high in protein but low in fat, such as skinless chicken and turkey, tuna packed in water, cod, ground turkey and low fat (1%) or skimmed milk.

I love junk food. Do I have to give it up completely?
You may have to forgo most junk food while you're pregnant. The foods we consider 'junk food' are usually high calorie, high fat foods that contain little nutrition for you or your baby. It's probably all right to eat junk food once in a while, but don't make it a regular part of your diet.

I've been craving certain foods now that I'm pregnant. Is this normal?
For many women, cravings during pregnancy are normal. Cravings for particular foods during pregnancy can be both good and bad. If you crave foods that are nutritious and healthy, eat them in moderate amounts. If you crave foods that are high in sugar and fat, and loaded with calories, be very careful about eating them.

Why do I have these cravings now, especially for foods that I might not normally eat?
No one knows for sure, but many believe it is because of the hormone changes and emotional changes that occur during pregnancy.

Some foods I normally love make me feel sick now. Why?
This is normal and very common during pregnancy. The hormones of pregnancy have a significant impact on the gastrointestinal tract, which can affect your reaction to certain foods.

I've heard bad things about artificial sweeteners during pregnancy. Are they really something to worry about?
Studies to date have not shown any harm to pregnancy from aspartame (Canderel). However, women who suffer from phenylketonuria need to follow a low-phenylalanine diet, or their babies may suffer from delayed development or even mental retardation. The phenylalanine in aspartame contributes to phenylalanine in your diet.

Saccharin is another artificial sweetener found in foods and beverages. It is still being tested for its effect on pregnancy. My advice with artificial sweeteners is to avoid them or use them in moderation during pregnancy.

I've found that I want to eat late at night, even though I've never felt hungry at night before. Should I eat late at night?

Late night nutritious snacks are beneficial for some women, especially if they must eat many small meals a day. However, many women should not snack at night because they don't need the extra calories. Food in the stomach late at night may also cause more distress if heartburn or nausea and vomiting are problems.

I'm 11 weeks pregnant and had my cholesterol checked last week. It was higher than the last time I had it checked. Is that normal?

Yes, Cholesterol levels usually increase during pregnancy and nursing because of hormone changes, so it's rather useless to have them tested at this time.

If feel so nauseated that I can't eat anything. Is this dangerous?

Nausea, also called *morning sickness*, is usually not dangerous because it doesn't last too long. It becomes dangerous when you are unable to eat an adequate amount of food or drink enough fluid. You should be able to eat nutritious foods even if you have morning sickness.

Nausea is typically at its worst during the beginning of pregnancy. It usually lessens and disappears late in the first trimester, and you will feel better for the rest of your pregnancy.

See Chapter 2 for further information about nausea and morning sickness.

My doctor told me to drink lots of water every day, but I hate it. Do I really need it?

Water is necessary for your body to process nutrients, develop new cells and sustain blood volume. You may also feel better if you drink more fluid than you normally do. Your blood volume increases during pregnancy; drinking extra fluids helps you keep up with this change.

How can drinking fluid help me?

Many women who suffer from headaches, uterine cramping and other problems during pregnancy find increasing their fluid intake helps resolve some of their symptoms. It also helps avoid bladder infections.

How much water do I need to drink?
Drink 3 pints (1.7 litres) of liquid every day. Water is the best liquid to choose. When your urine is light yellow to clear, you're getting enough water. Dark yellow urine is a sign that you need to add more fluid to your diet.

If I drink beverages that normally act as diuretics, will it counteract the increase in fluids?
No, it will not.

How can I possibly drink this much extra fluid?
It's really not that hard. Some women drink water, one glass at a time, throughout the day. (Decrease your intake later in the day so you don't have to go to the bathroom all night long.)

My husband and I eat out a lot because we're tired after work. Are there any foods I should avoid at restaurants?
It's all right to eat out at restaurants; you just need to be a little more careful about what you eat. Avoid any raw meats or raw seafood such as sushi. You may also find that certain foods do not agree with you, so avoid those foods.

What foods should I choose at a restaurant?
Fish, fresh vegetables and salads are usually your best bets, but be careful with calorie-loaded salad dressings if excessive weight gain is a concern. Avoid highly spicy foods or foods that contain a lot of sodium, such as some Chinese food. You may experience water retention after eating these foods.

I drink a few cups of coffee and several glasses of diet cola every day. Do I need to worry about caffeine?
Drinking as few as 4 cups of coffee a day (800mg of caffeine) by a pregnant woman has been said to be associated with decreased birth weight and a smaller head size in the newborn.

Although an exact 'toxic' amount for caffeine has not been determined, it makes sense to limit your caffeine intake.

What foods contain caffeine?
Caffeine is found in many beverages and foods, including coffee, tea, cola drinks and chocolate. Some medicines, such as cough medicines

and headache medicines also contain a lot of caffeine. It's important to read the labels.

Why is caffeine a problem?
Caffeine stimulates the central nervous system. There are no known benefits from caffeine for you or your unborn fetus. Caffeine can also affect calcium metabolism in both you and your baby.

What do you suggest about caffeine intake in pregnancy?
Limit your caffeine intake during pregnancy and if you breast feed. Read labels on foods, beverages and non-prescription medicines to find out about caffeine. Eliminate caffeine from your diet as much as possible.

Is that any place I can get more information on nutrition while I'm pregnant?
Ask your doctor or midwife.

Vitamins and Minerals

Do I really need to take antenatal vitamins?
Yes. Antenatal vitamins contain the recommended daily amounts of vitamins and minerals you need during pregnancy. They are taken to ensure your health and your baby's health. However, they aren't a substitute for food or a good diet.

How are antenatal vitamins different from other vitamins?
The main different between antenatal vitamins and regular vitamins is that antenatal vitamins also contain iron and folic acid supplements.

Do I need mineral supplements during my pregnancy?
The only material that needs to be supplemented during pregnancy is iron. The average woman's diet seldom contains enough iron to meet the increased demands of pregnancy. Your blood volume increases by 50 per cent in a normal pregnancy, and iron is an important part of blood production in your body.

I've heard I might have to take iron supplements during pregnancy. Does it really make a difference if I don't take an iron supplement?
Antenatal vitamins contain some iron but you may need to take extra iron. One of the first tests your doctor does is for anaemia. If he or she determines that you need an iron supplement, you must take it for your health and that of your baby.

How much iron is there in antenatal vitamins?
Most antenatal vitamins contain 60mg of elemental iron.

Won't iron make me constipated?
Constipation can be a side effect of taking iron. Work with your doctor to find the correct amount of iron to avoid side effects.

Will my baby have healthier teeth (when he or she gets them!) if I take extra fluoride during my pregnancy?
The use of fluoride and fluoride supplements during pregnancy is controversial. Some researchers believe fluoride supplements during pregnancy result in improved teeth in your child, but not everyone agrees. However, no harm to the baby has been shown from fluoride supplements in a pregnant woman. Some antenatal vitamins contain fluoride.

I've heard I should avoid sodium during pregnancy. What is it?
Sodium is a chemical that works to maintain the proper amount of fluid in your body. During pregnancy it can also affect your baby's system. Sodium is found in salty foods (such as potato crisps and dill pickles) and in processed foods, from soups to meats. You need *some* sodium; you just don't need too much of it. Read food labels to discover just how much you are getting!

How much sodium should I take in each day?
During pregnancy, keep your consumption of sodium under 3g (3,000mg) a day.

How can too much sodium hurt me or my baby?
Too much sodium is believed by some doctors to cause water retention, swelling and high blood pressure. Any of these can be a problem for you.

Sodium Content of Some Foods

Fresh or Minimally Prepared Foods

8oz (240ml) apple juice	2mg
3 apricots (fresh)	1mg
1 medium banana	1mg
8oz (240g) fish	170mg
1 head lettuce	15mg
1 medium carrot	35mg
1 large egg	70mg
8oz (240g) green beans (frozen)	2mg
3oz (90g) minced beef	60mg
1 lemon	1mg
8oz (240ml) whole milk	120mg
8oz (240g) oatmeal (long-cooked)	10mg
8oz (240ml) orange juice	2mg
1 peach	1mg
3oz (90g) pork	65mg

Prepared Foods

3oz (90g) bacon	1,400mg
8oz (240g) baked beans	100mg
1 slice white bread	100mg
1 frozen chicken dinner	1,400mg
8oz (240ml) chicken noodle soup	1,050mg
1 cinnamon roll	630mg
1 tablespoonful cooking oil	0mg
3oz (90g) corned beef	1,500mg
8oz (240g) cornflakes	305mg
8oz (240g) green beans	320mg
8oz (240g) plain flour	2mg
8oz (240g) self-raising flour	1,565mg
1 tablespoonful Italian dressing	250mg
1 tablespoonful ketchup	155mg
1 olive	165mg
1 dill pickle	1,930mg
8oz (240g) pudding, instant	335mg
8oz (240g) puffed rice cereal	1mg
8oz (240ml) tomato juice	640mg

Fast Foods

1 turkey sandwich	1,060mg
1 Burger King Whopper	675mg
1 hotdog	990mg
1 chicken dinner (3 pieces)	2,285mg
1 McDonald's Big Mac	1,010mg

I don't know what foods contain sodium. What should I avoid?
You can't avoid something unless you know where to find it. With sodium, that can be tricky. It's in the salt shaker and in salty-tasting foods, such as pretzels, chips and salted nuts. You may be surprised by the amount of sodium in foods that *don't* taste salty.

Sodium is found in canned and processed products, fast foods, cereals, desserts and even soft drinks and some medicines. See the chart on the previous page for a listing of the sodium content in a variety of foods. Read the labels!

Exercise

I love to exercise and don't want to stop while I'm pregnant. Do I have to?
Experts agree that exercise during pregnancy is safe and beneficial for most pregnant women, if it is done properly. This is definitely an area to discuss with your doctor at the beginning of your pregnancy!

I don't really like to exercise, but I do it. Are there benefits to continuing my exercise programme during my pregnancy?
Regular, moderate exercise during pregnancy can be beneficial for you in many ways. It can help:

• relieve backache
• prevent constipation and varicose veins
• strengthen muscles needed for delivery
• leave you in better shape after delivery
• help you feel better

What should my exercise goals be during pregnancy?
The goal of exercising during pregnancy is overall good health. It will make you feel better physically, and it can give you an emotional boost.

My mother told me I shouldn't exercise during pregnancy; she was warned not to when she was pregnant with me. Why the change now?
Exercise was not always approved for a pregnant woman. In the past, doctors were concerned about the redirection of blood flow from the fetus to the mother-to-be's muscles during exercise. We now know this occurs to a small degree, but it is not harmful to the fetus in a normal pregnancy.

I've never exercised before, but I'd like to begin now. Can I?
Some women become interested in exercising during pregnancy to help them feel better. If you've never exercised before, you *must* discuss it with your doctor before you begin. Pregnancy is *not* the time to begin a vigorous exercise programme.

What kind of exercises will my doctor recommend?
If you've never exercised before, walking and swimming are excellent forms of exercise. Riding a stationary bike can also be enjoyable.

I want to exercise, and it scares me that I might do something to hurt my pregnancy. Should I be scared?
It's a good idea to be fit and to exercise when you're pregnant. If you're fit, you'll do better with weight gain during pregnancy, be able to do the work of labour and delivery better, and feel better after the birth. Exercise during pregnancy isn't without risks, including increased body temperature, decreased blood flow to the uterus and possible injury to you.

Most experts recommend reducing your exercise to 70–80 per cent of your prepregnancy level. If you have problems with bleeding or cramping or have had problem pregnancies before, you will need to modify your exercise with your doctor's advice.

Someone told me exercising can cause early labour. Should I believe her?
It was once believed that exercise could cause preterm labour because there is a temporary increase in uterine activity following exercise. However, in a normal pregnancy, this does not cause a problem.

I read that my baby's heart rate increases when mine does during exercise. Can this cause a problem?
The fetal heart rate increases somewhat during and immediately after exercise, but it stays within the normal fetal range of 120–160 beats a minute. This should not cause any problems for you or the baby.

My aerobics instructor said my heart rate changes during pregnancy. Why?
During pregnancy, your heart rate is higher so you don't have to exercise as vigorously to reach your target heart rate range. Be careful not to stress your cardiovascular system.

What if my heart rate is too high?
If it's too high, slow down but don't stop exercising completely. Continue exercising but at a more moderate rate.

What if my pulse rate is too low?
If you don't feel too winded, pick up the pace a bit, but don't overdo it. Check your pulse rate again in a few minutes to make sure you aren't overexerting yourself.

How often should I check my pulse rate?
During pregnancy, you should do this fairly often. It will surprise you how fast your pulse can increase during a pregnancy workout.

I'm not sure how I figure out my heart rate. Can you explain it?
While you are pregnant, your pulse rate should not exceed 120 beats per minute for more than 15 minutes during a workout. Check your pulse with the following steps.

- Have a clock with a second hand in view.
- Place the index and middle fingers of one hand on the side of your neck where you can feel your pulse.
- After finding your pulse, watch the second hand until it reaches the 12.
- Begin counting the pulse beats until the second hand reaches the 2 (10 seconds).
- Multiply that number by 6 to find your heart rate.

When should I consult my doctor about exercising during pregnancy?
Discuss it with him or her at your *first* antenatal visit. If you decide later to start or to change your exercise programme, be sure to consult your physician before you begin. Some women should *not* exercise during pregnancy. If you experience any of the following symptoms, do *not* exercise during your pregnancy:

- a history of an incompetent cervix, preterm labour or repeated miscarriages
- high blood pressure early in pregnancy
- multiple fetuses (twins, triplets or more)
- diagnosed heart disease
- pre-eclampsia
- vaginal bleeding

Will I have to change my exercise programme during pregnancy?
Changes in your body due to pregnancy will cause you to change the
way you exercise. Your centre of gravity changes, so you will need to
adjust your exercise for that. As your abdomen grows larger, you will
find you can't do some activities very comfortably and you may have
to stop others altogether.

*I feel out of breath more quickly when I exercise now that I'm
pregnant. is something wrong with me?*
Your growing abdomen can put a strain on your respiratory system,
causing you to feel out of breath sooner than normal. When you
exercise, don't work to the point that you cannot talk and have trouble
breathing. This indicates that you are working too strenuously; cut
back on your workout.

I feel a lot hotter when I exercise during pregnancy. Is this normal?
When you're pregnant, you normally feel warmer than usual. You'll
feel warmer, too, when you exercise, so try to avoid becoming
overheated during workouts. Work out in a well-ventilated room, and
drink lots of water while you exercise.

*I'm 9 weeks pregnant and haven't exercised for years. Can I start
now?*
It is possible to start exercising now, but begin gradually. It's best to
discuss your desire to exercise with your doctor *before* you begin any
programme. If you don't have any problems with your pregnancy, you
should be able to exercise as long as you are comfortable. The key is
not to try to do too much too fast. The best exercises for you are
walking and swimming.

Can I play competitive sports during pregnancy?
If you are used to playing a competitive sport, such as tennis, you
should be able to continue, but expect to reduce the level of
competition. The point to remember is not to get carried away or to
overwork yourself.

What are some good sports to do while I'm pregnant?
Some of the less strenuous sports are listed below. Most are generally
considered safe for a normal, low risk pregnancy.

- walking
- swimming
- low impact aerobics designed especially for pregnancy
- water aerobics
- stationary bicycling
- regular cycling (if you're experienced)
- jogging (if you jogged before pregnancy)
- tennis (played moderately)

What sports should I avoid during pregnancy?

The sports listed below should be avoided during pregnancy because of the potential problems associated with each:

- scuba diving
- water skiing
- surfing
- horse riding
- downhill or cross-country skiing
- any contact sport

My health club offers aerobics classes for pregnant women. Are these better than the regular aerobics classes?

Aerobics classes specifically designed for pregnant women are a good choice. They concentrate on the unique needs of the pregnant woman, such as strengthening abdominal muscles and improving posture. When choosing a class, be sure the instructor has proper training and check with your doctor.

If I exercise, do I need to eat more?

Your nutrition needs increase during pregnancy, and you do burn extra calories during exercise, so you should consume enough calories to ensure a balanced diet. As I've already discussed, a woman of normal weight before pregnancy needs to eat between 300 and 800 extra calories a day during pregnancy. Exercising may require you to eat more.

Will exercise during pregnancy make labour and delivery easier?

Exercise during pregnancy should help you have an easier time with your labour and delivery.

Will exercise help me recover more quickly after my baby is born?
Many believe that women who exercise during pregnancy have a shorter recovery time after birth. Exercise keeps you fit so you can get back in shape more quickly.

Can you give me more guidelines about exercising during pregnancy?
As I've stated, be sure you consult with your doctor before you begin any exercise programme. Follow the tips below to keep you healthy and in good shape.

- Try to exercise at least 3 times a week for 20–30 minutes each time.
- Start your exercise routine with 5 minutes of warm-up and end with a 5-minute cool-down period.
- Wear comfortable clothes that offer support. Wear a support bra and good athletics shoes.
- Drink plenty of water during exercise.
- Don't exercise strenuously for more than 15–20 minutes.
- Check your pulse rate; keep it below 120 beats a minute.
- Don't exercise in hot, humid weather.
- After the fourth month of pregnancy, avoid exercises that require you to lie on your back.
- Never allow your body temperature to rise above 100.4°F (38°C).
- Stop immediately and consult your physician if you experience any problems.

What kind of problems should I watch out for while I'm exercising?
Be aware of any unusual occurrences, and report them to your doctor immediately. Be careful about the following:

- pain
- bleeding
- dizziness
- extreme shortness of breath
- heart palpitations
- faintness
- abnormally rapid heart rate
- back pain
- pubic pain
- difficulty walking

Weight Management

I'm in good shape; I exercise regularly and my weight is about where it should be. How much weight should I gain during my pregnancy?
Normal weight gain during pregnancy is 24–28lb (11–13kg). This may sound like a lot, but if you add up weight for the baby, placenta, amniotic fluid and changes in you, it really isn't that much. See the chart on the opposite page for general guidelines to weight gain during pregnancy.

How am I supposed to watch my weight gain and still eat 300–800 calories more a day?
Not every woman needs to increase her food intake by 300–800 calories; that's just a general guideline. You must look at your individual case. If you are underweight when you begin pregnancy, you may have to eat *more* than 800 extra calories each day. If you're overweight when you get pregnant, you may have less need for extra calories.

I believe the key to good nutrition and weight management is to eat a balanced diet throughout your entire pregnancy. Eat the foods you need to help your baby grow and develop, but choose wisely. For example, if you're overweight, avoid peanut butter and other nuts as a protein source; choose water-packed tuna or low fat cheeses instead. If you're underweight, select ice cream and milkshakes as sources of dairy foods.

I have such a fear of getting fat during pregnancy, I know it's going to cause me a lot of problems. What can I do about it?
You must be prepared to gain weight while you're pregnant. It is a normal part of pregnancy, and it is necessary for your baby's health! Getting on the scales and seeing your weight increase can be hard for some women, especially those who have to watch their weight closely. You must decide at the beginning of your pregnancy that it is all right to gain weight – it's for the health of your baby. You can control your weight gain by eating carefully and nutritiously; you don't have to gain an extra 50lb (22.5kg). But you must gain enough weight to meet the needs of pregnancy.

General Weight Gain Guidelines for Pregnancy

Current Weight	Acceptable Gain
Underweight	26–35lb 12–16kg
Normal weight	24–28lb 11–13kg
Overweight	15–22lb 7–10kg

When my mother was pregnant with me, she was allowed to gain just 13lb (5.85kg) for her entire pregnancy. Was that normal 35 years ago?

Yes, it was fairly normal then. We have learned a lot about pregnancy because of advances in technology and information from research and other sources. We realise today that it is permissible and advisable for a women to gain a sufficient amount of weight during pregnancy; today the normal weight gain during pregnancy is 24–28lb (11–13kg) – quite a change from 13lb (5.85kg)!

I'm pregnant, and know I'm underweight. How much should I gain during my pregnancy?

If you start your pregnancy underweight, the normal weight gain is 26–35lb (12–16kg). It is important for you to eat regularly and to eat nutritiously, even if you are not used to doing this.

I'm overweight, and I have just found out I'm pregnant. How much weight should I gain while I'm pregnant?

If you're overweight before pregnancy, you probably should not gain as much as other women during your pregnancy. Acceptable weight gain is 15–22lb (7–10kg). This is an individual problem that you should discuss with your doctor. It is important for you to eat nutritious, well-balanced meals during your pregnancy. Do *not* diet!

How much should I gain each week during pregnancy?

As an average for a normal weight woman, some doctors suggest 10oz (300g) a week until 20 weeks, then 1lb (450g) a week from 20 to 40 weeks. However, this varies for each woman. If you're concerned, talk to your doctor about it.

I'm 7 weeks pregnant and haven't gained any weight; I think I may even have lost 2–3lb (0.9–1.35kg). Is that all right?
It isn't unusual not to gain weight or even to lose a little weight early in pregnancy. Your doctor or midwife will keep track of the change in your weight during your pregnancy.

My doctor said I must be weighed each time I come in. Can't I just weigh myself at home before I come in and tell the doctor or nurse my weight?
It's best to be weighed at the antenatal clinic. It is one way your doctor can tell that everything is progressing normally with your pregnancy. Although you may be shy about being weighed, it's an important part of your visit to the doctor. Your health care team is doing it to make sure everything is all right with your pregnancy.

My friend told me I should gain about 18–28lb (8–13kg) with my pregnancy. That sounds like a lot to me when the baby only weighs about 7lb (3kg) Where does all that weight go?
Your friend is right. The weight that you gain is distributed as shown in the chart below. As you can see, some weight will be lost during the birth process. More weight is often lost as your body readjusts to its non-pregnant state.

Distribution of Weight gained during Pregnancy

Weight	Location
7½lb (3.4kg)	Baby
4lb (1.8kg)	Increased fluid volume
2lb (0.9kg)	Uterus
2lb (0.9kg)	Amniotic fluid
2lb (0.9kg)	Breast enlargement
1½lb (0.7kg)	Placenta

CHAPTER 6

Fatigue, Work and Pregnancy

I have just found out I'm pregnant. I'm so tired all the time. Is it normal for a pregnant woman to feel so exhausted?
Pregnancy can cause you to feel extremely tired. Fatigue is normal and common, and may continue during your entire pregnancy. For most women, it is at its worst early in pregnancy, then gets better. Eating well, taking vitamins and getting plenty of rest will help. We know pregnant women need more sleep than they normally would. In most cases, 8–10 hours of sleep at night will help you feel better. When you see your doctor, one of the first tests he or she will do is a haemoglobin test to check for anaemia, which can also be a reason for feeling tired.

My sister said it's not good for me to lie on my back during pregnancy. Does she know what she's talking about?
It *is* best for you not to lie on your back when you sleep or rest. As your uterus grows, lying on your back can place the uterus on top of important blood vessels (*inferior vena cava* and *aorta*) that run down the back of your abdomen. This can decrease circulation to your baby and to parts of your body. It may also be harder for you to breathe when you lie on your back.

I usually lie on my stomach when I sleep. Will I be able to do this as I get bigger?
Lying on your stomach when you sleep or rest isn't a good idea. It puts a lot of pressure on your growing uterus, which will become a comfort problem later. The bigger you get, the harder it is to lie on your stomach.

What is the best position for sleeping?
Learn to sleep on your side – you'll be glad you did as you get bigger. Use some extra pillows to support your back so you don't lie flat. Rest your top leg on another pillow. A 'pregnancy pillow' that provides support for your entire body may help.

I've been under a lot of stress during my pregnancy. Is there anything I can do to help me manage the stress better?
The following breathing exercise can help you relax when you feel stressed:

- Inhale slowly as you count to 4. Push your abdomen out as you breathe in.
- Let your shoulders and neck relax as you slowly exhale while counting to 6.
- Repeat as often as you need to.

Hint Play gentle, soothing background music when you practise this exercise.

I've heard that there are exercises to do to help relieve stress. Can you tell me about them?
One exercise I recommend to my patients is to relax each muscle group with each deep breath. Start with the feet and work up through the legs, hands, arms, torso, shoulders, neck and face. Continue for 10–20 minutes. This exercise also works when you're lying in bed and are having trouble getting to sleep.

As my pregnancy progresses, I find that I'm having trouble getting comfortable. What should I do?
If you're having trouble sleeping, experiment with different positions when you rest. Lie on your side, with a pillow under your abdomen. Elevate your feet to help keep blood moving throughout your body, especially your legs. Or you might feel better if you elevate your head and shoulders.

I can't sleep enough at night to make me feel better. How do I get the rest I need?
Try taking naps during the day. If you can't nap, sit down and relax – listen to music or read, if that helps. When you relax, prop your feet above your chest if possible, to help with swelling and to ease discomfort in your legs.

Working during Pregnancy

My mother told me I shouldn't work during pregnancy. Is this true?
In the past, women were encouraged or even forced to stop working when they were pregnant. Today, many women work until they deliver their baby. Whether you work for your entire pregnancy depends on your particular circumstances. If you are concerned about it, discuss it with your doctor.

My husband is concerned about my working during my pregnancy. Should he be?
More than half of all women work outside the home; many pregnant women work and do well. If you are concerned about whether your job is safe for your pregnancy, discuss your particular situation with your doctor. It may be difficult to know the specific risk of a particular job – the goal is to minimise the risk to you and your baby while still enabling you to work. A normal, healthy woman should be able to work at most jobs throughout her pregnancy.

Can my work be hazardous to my pregnancy?
Certain factors may increase the risk from working during your pregnancy. If your job includes two or more of the following, discuss it with your doctor. He or she may want to monitor your pregnancy more closely.

- prolonged standing (more than 3 hours a day)
- work on an industrial machine, especially if it vibrates a great deal or requires strenuous effort to operate it
- strenuous physical tasks, such as heavy lifting or heavy cleaning
- repetitious, tedious work, such as assembly-line jobs
- environmental factors, such as high noise levels or extreme temperatures
- long working hours
- shift changes

I don't want to stop working while I'm pregnant. What precautions should I take?
You will probably have to slow down if you continue to work. You may also have to take it a little easier; you may not be able to do some of the things you do when you are not pregnant. It may also be necessary to ask for help in some of the tasks you are required to perform.

Should I try to rest during my working day?

If possible, try to lie down during breaks or in your lunch hour. Even sitting down in a quiet place can be beneficial. Ten or 15 minutes of rest can make you feel better and restore your energy.

A colleague who has just had a baby said her doctor told her she should exercise her legs and feet often during the day while she was pregnant. Should I do the same?

Yes. Try to do some leg-stretching foot exercises several times each hour. Sit down and remove your shoes before doing the following exercise. Extend your legs in front, then point your toes and flex your feet. Repeat this four or five times. It helps circulation in your feet and may prevent some swelling in your legs.

I've heard I should wear maternity tights to work. Why?

Whether you sit or stand at work, maternity tights provide support for your legs. They can be helpful, even if you don't work. Maternity tights may be preferable to ordinary support tights because they don't constrict your waist or abdomen. If you are concerned, discuss it with your doctor.

My job require me to stand all day. Will that be a problem?

Studies show that women who stand all day have smaller babies. If you stand all day, you may have problems at the end of your pregnancy with swelling of your feet and ankles. It may be necessary for you to modify your work or to be able to lie down a couple of times during the day or to work fewer hours.

I have to climb a lot in my job. Should I talk to my supervisor about it?

It's probably best to avoid activities that involve climbing and balance in your job, especially during the third trimester. Talk with your supervisor about eliminating these activities.

I seem to have terrible mood swings while I'm at the office. Is this normal?

Elevated hormones can trigger mood swings in you. You may also find you're more tired; it's normal. Take a break if any situation becomes more than you can bear.

I know my centre of gravity is changing. What's the best way for me to lift an object?
Do most of your lifting with your legs. Bend your knees to lift; don't bend at the waist. As your abdomen grows larger, don't lift anything over 30lb (13.6kg).

I work at a computer terminal all day long, and I've heard that this can harm my baby. Is it true?
To date, we have no evidence that working at a computer terminal can harm a growing baby. However, if you work at one, you should be aware of how long you sit and the way you sit. See the next question.

I have a job that keeps me sitting behind a desk all day. Is there anything I need to be concerned about?
If you have a 'sit-down' job, it's probably best to get up and move around regularly to stimulate your circulation. Take short walks frequently. Sit in a chair that offers good support for your back and legs. Don't slouch or cross your legs while sitting. Make sure you get up and walk around every 15 minutes.

I read that some substances or conditions in the workplace can harm a developing baby. What are they?
According to Maureen Paul MD MPH, Director of the Occupational Reproductive Hazards Center at the University of Massachusetts in the US, some substances can cause harm to a developing fetus. The chart on the next page describes various agents, their sources and the possible effects they may have on a growing baby.

Is there a danger that my partner or I could bring home traces of substances we are exposed to at work?
Yes. Substances may be brought into your home on your work clothes or the work clothes of someone else in your family. If you think you may be exposed to hazardous substances, be sure to discuss it with your doctor.

Workplace Hazards and Possible Effects on the Fetus

Agent	Sources	Possible Effects
Cytomegalovirus	Hospitals, day-care centres	Congenital malformation
Cytotoxic drugs	Hospital or pharmacy preparation of chemotherapeutic drugs	Miscarriage
Ethylene oxide	Surgical instrument sterilisation	Miscarriage
Ionising radiation	X-rays and radiation treatments, radioactive implants, nuclear power plants	In very high doses, congenital malformation; lower doses may increase childhood cancer risk
Lead	House, car and art paints made before 1980; battery manufacturing plants and radiator repair shops; ceramics and glass manufacturers; toll booths on heavily used roads	Preterm birth, delayed development of intelligence
Organic solvents	Paint thinners, lacquers, adhesives; electronics and printing plants	Congenital malformation
PCBs (polychlorinated biphenyls)	Electronic capacitors and transformers; hazardous waste industry	Delayed development of intelligence
Rubella virus	Day-care centres, schools	Congenital malformation
Toxoplasmosis	Veterinary clinics, animal shelters, meat-packing operations	Congenital malformation

You and Your Rights

I work full time and am worried I may lose my job because I am pregnant. Am I entitled to maternity leave?
Since October 1994, as a working mother-to-be, you are entitled to maternity leave, protection against unfair dismissal for pregnancy-related reasons and protection against any risks to your health and safety in the workplace.

Every woman who is in work while she is pregnant is entitled to 14 weeks' maternity leave. When you return to work you will go back to the same job. This right applies to every employee who gives the required notice, with no requirement about number of hours you work or length of time you have worked for the employer.

Write to your employer at least 21 days before you start your maternity leave, telling him or her you are pregnant and giving the expected date of childbirth. If circumstances (for example, illness) prevent you from giving 21 days' notice, you must write to your employer as soon as you can. You must also say the date you intend to start your maternity leave, but you only need to put this in writing if your employer requests it. If requested you must also enclose a copy of your maternity certificate (form MAT BI; in Northern Ireland, MBI) which your midwife or doctor can give you when you are about 24 weeks pregnant.

Will I be able to take time off from work for antenatal appointments?
Yes. This is your right and includes attendance at relaxation classes and parentcraft classes, including travelling time, without losing any pay. Your employer may wish to have a letter from your doctor or midwife saying that classes are part of your antenatal care.

You should let your employer know when you will need to attend antenatal appointments and he or she may wish for confirmation that you did attend.

If you are refused time off or are not paid you can make a claim within 3 months to a industrial tribunal.

When can I start maternity leave?
The earliest you can start is 11 weeks before the baby is due. It's up to you to decide when you want to stop work. You can work right up to the week of expected childbirth. The exception is if in the last 11 weeks of pregnancy you have a pregnancy-related illness and are away even for one day. You may be asked to start your maternity leave.

If I take maternity leave will I retain my contractual rights?

During the 14 weeks of maternity leave you will retain your rights to holiday entitlement, pension rights, and company car, but you will only get maternity pay (see below).

Do I have to give notice of return to work?

Not if you are going back at the end of your 14 weeks' maternity leave. If you want to return to work before that you must give your employer 7 days' notice in writing. Otherwise, if you just return, your employer can send you away for 7 days, or until the end of your 14 weeks' leave, whichever is the sooner.

You are not allowed to work for 2 weeks after delivery of the baby so if your pregnancy goes overdue and your maternity leave runs out it will be extended to 2 weeks after the delivery.

If you are ill at the end of your maternity leave and unable to return to work, you should obtain a medical certificate to give your employer. You should be able to get your pay from him or her and if he or she gets the certificate before your maternity leave is over you will be protected from unfair dismissal for an additional 4 weeks.

What is Extended Maternity Absence?

You may qualify for this if you have worked for the same employer for two years by the time you are 28 weeks pregnant, you work until you are 12 weeks pregnant, and you work for a firm which employs more than 5 people.

Extended maternity absence can last for up to 29 weeks after the baby is born. You must give your employer written notice, 21 days before you start your maternity leave, that you intend to take extended leave after your baby is delivered but intend to return to work at the end of this time.

Your employer may ask you, after 11 weeks of maternity leave, to confirm that you intend to return to work and you must reply within 10 days, notifying him or her of your intended date of return to work.

After that you can only delay returning to work on the day you have notified if you are ill, or the employer wishes to delay your return for up to 4 weeks for a specified reason, if there is a strike, or if your employer agrees.

What do I do if my employer tries to dismiss me or select me for redundancy for a reason connected with pregnancy, childbirth or maternity leave?

This is against the law. Your employer must give you a statement of the reasons for dismissal. If you believe dismissal is related to the pregnancy you need advice from a trade union or a Citizens' Advice Bureau about putting in a claim to the industrial tribunal within 3 months. You may need to involve a solicitor.

What do I do if I think my working conditions are putting my health or my baby's health at risk?

If you are pregnant, have given birth within the last 6 months, or are breast feeding, your employer must not allow this. You must notify your employer of your condition in writing. He or she is required to carry out a risk assessment in your workplace and to comply with any obligations specified in health and safety regulations. If work conditions still put your health or your baby's at risk, your employer must change the working conditions or offer you a suitable alternative job. If he or she can't do this he or she must suspend you on full pay, but if you unreasonably refuse alternative work you lose your right to full pay during suspension. If you do night work your doctor may advise this is unsuitable and you then have the right to transfer to day work or be suspended on full pay.

If you are refused any of these rights you should consult a trade union or a solicitor.

Maternity Pay and Benefits

What is Statutory Maternity Pay?

A weekly payment for a maximum of 18 weeks starting when you leave work, even if you do not plan to go back to work. The earliest you can start to be paid is at 29 weeks pregnant (unless you have an intra-uterine death of the fetus, when you can start at 24 weeks if this occurs). If you have a pregnancy-related illness in the last 6 weeks your maternity pay will start then. If your illness is not pregnancy related you can claim Statutory Sick Pay until your maternity leave starts.

Your employer will pay your Statutory Maternity Pay on a weekly or monthly basis according to how your salary is normally paid, and income tax and National Insurance will be deducted.

Who is eligible for Statutory Maternity Pay?

You must have worked for the same employer for at least 26 weeks before you are 25 weeks pregnant and still be in work by then; you must be earning at least £59 per week (1996).

How much is Statutory Maternity Pay?

For the first 6 weeks you get 90 per cent of your average pay. After this you get £54.55 weekly for up to 12 weeks.

How do I get Statutory Maternity Pay?

Write to your employer at least 3 weeks before you stop work, and send him or her a copy of your maternity certificate (form MAT BI, or MBI in Northern Ireland), which you can obtain from your midwife or family doctor.

What is a Maternity Allowance?

This is a weekly allowance for women who are not eligible for Statutory Maternity Pay. You can obtain the allowance if you are self-employed, if you gave up work, or if you changed jobs during your pregnancy. You must have paid National Insurance for at least 26 of the 66 weeks before the week in which the baby is due. (Check with your local social security office to see if you qualify.)

The lower rate of £47.35 (1996) a week is paid to women who are either self-employed or unemployed in the qualifying week (the 25th week of pregnancy). A higher rate of £54.55 (1996) a week is paid to women who are employed in the qualifying week.

To claim, you must obtain a form MAI from your antenatal clinic or social security office (Incapacity Benefit Branch in Northern Ireland) and send them the completed form as soon as you can after 26 weeks of pregnancy.

What is Incapacity Benefit?

If you can't get Statutory Maternity Pay or a Maternity Allowance, but have worked and paid National Insurance in the last 3 years, you may be able to get this benefit (£46.15 a week in 1996). You claim on the same form (MAI) as soon as you can after 26 weeks. Your social security office will check if you can receive Incapacity Benefit. Your maternity certificate (form MAT BI; or MBI in Northern Ireland) should be submitted with the claim.

CHAPTER 7

More than One Baby!

How does a multiple pregnancy occur?
The babies may come from a single egg that divides after fertilisation, or more than one egg may be fertilised.

How frequent are twins?
Twins from one egg occur about once in every 250 births around the world. Twins from two eggs occur in 1 out of every 100 births in white women and in 1 out of 79 births in black women. In certain areas in Africa, twins occur once in every 20 births! The occurrence of twins in Oriental population is less common – about 1 in every 150 births.

My doctor has told me she thinks I may be carrying triplets. How common are they?
Triplets are not very common; they occur only once in every 8,000 deliveries. Many doctors never deliver a set of triplets in their entire career!

I have heard the incidence of twins is on the increase. Why is that?
Researchers believe two factors are responsible for this increase. One is the wider use of fertility drugs, which can result in multiple births. The second is the growing number of women who are having babies at an older age. We know the chance of twins increases as a woman gets older.

How do fertility drugs cause an increase in the rate of twins?
Fertility drugs can stimulate the ovaries to release more than one egg, increasing the chance of a multiple pregnancy.

Why do older women have a greater chance of having twins?
The incidence of twins is highest among women between ages 35 and 39. This increase has been attributed to higher levels of *gonadotropin*, the hormone that stimulates the ovaries to develop and release eggs. As a woman gets older, the level of gonadotropin increases, and she is more likely to produce two eggs during one menstrual cycle.

What is the difference between identical and fraternal twins?
Identical (or *monozygotic*) *twins* develop from a single egg that divides after being fertilised. Babies are always the same sex, and they look alike. When two eggs are fertilised, the babies will be as different in appearance as any other brothers and sisters. They are called *fraternal* or *dizygotic twins*.

Are most twins born to older women fraternal twins?
Usually that is the case. Because babies are born from two different eggs, they are fraternal (not identical).

I've heard that twin births can run in families. Is this true?
Yes, on the *mother's* side. One study showed that if a woman was a twin, the chance of her giving birth to twins was about 1 in 58! If a woman is the daughter of a twin, she also has a higher chance of having twins. Another study reported that 1 out of 24 twins' mothers (4 per cent) was also a twin, but only 1 out of 60 (1.7 per cent) of the fathers was a twin.

I read that the more children a woman has, the more likely she is to have twins. Does this really happen?
Yes, it does. Research has proved that a woman has a greater chance of having twins the more pregnancies she has. I know of one woman who had three single births, then twins, then triplets!

A friend told me about her sister-in-law, who was told early in pregnancy she was going to have twins. Then sometime later, one of the twins disappeared. Is she making this up?
No, this has happened. Early ultrasound examinations have revealed two babies; later ultrasounds of the same woman showed that one baby had disappeared, but the other baby was all right. We believe one of the fetuses may die, then be absorbed in the mother's body. This is one reason many doctors prefer not to predict a twin birth before 10 weeks of pregnancy.

Someone said twins are more common with in vitro fertilisation. Why?
This is because more than one embryo is replaced inside the woman's body so as to increase her chances of having a baby. It's also interesting to note that more girls than boys are born to women who undergo in vitro fertilisation (fertilisation outside the body).

When is a twin pregnancy most often discovered?
A twin pregnancy is usually found during the second trimester because the woman is larger than expected and growth seems to be too fast.

What's the best way to diagnose a multiple pregnancy?
Ultrasound scanning is the best way to see if a woman is carrying more than one baby.

If a woman is pregnant with more than one baby, is she likely to have more problems during pregnancy?
The possibility of problems does increase slightly when a woman is carrying more than one baby. Possible problems include:

- increased miscarriage
- fetal death or mortality
- fetal malformations
- low birth weight or growth retardation
- pre-eclampsia

Ultrasound scan of three fetuses (triplets) early in pregnancy.

- maternal anaemia
- problems with the placenta
- maternal bleeding or haemorrhage
- problems with the umbilical cords
- hydramnios or polyhydramnios (too much fluid in the bag of waters)
- labour complicated by breech or transverse presentation
- premature labour

If I'm expecting more than one baby, what do I have to keep in mind during my pregnancy?

One of the most important things you must remember with a multiple pregnancy is to take things more slowly, from the beginning of your pregnancy until delivery. Taking care of yourself is the best way to take care of your developing babies.

Is it true that a woman who is carrying more than one baby needs to eat more?

It is necessary for a woman who is carrying more than one baby to eat more – at least 300 more calories *per baby* each day than in a single pregnancy! A woman needs more protein, minerals, vitamins and essential fatty acids. Iron supplementation is also necessary.

I recently read an article about 'conjoined twins'. What are they?

Conjoined twins, until recently also called *Siamese twins*, are twins whose bodies are connected at some point. It is a very serious complication of pregnancy because these babies may share important internal organs, such as the heart, lungs or liver. Sometimes they can be separated; often they cannot.

How are conjoined twins delivered?

It is usually necessary to deliver conjoined twins by caesarean section.

Does the birth of conjoined twins occur very often?

No, it is very rare.

Will I have a greater chance of having iron-deficiency anaemia if I have twins?

Often women who are pregnant with more than one baby do have iron-deficiency anaemia. A multiple pregnancy is more stressful for your body than a single pregnancy, and your needs increase in many areas.

Can I exercise during pregnancy if I'm expecting twins?

As a general rule, we advise women who are carrying more than one baby *not* to exercise during pregnancy because of the extra stress with which their bodies will be dealing.

I'd like to try to keep in shape during pregnancy. What exercises can I do?

Walking and swimming *may* be permissible for you while you're pregnant with multiple fetuses. Be sure to check out any exercise programme with your doctor before you start it . However, do not do anything that is strenuous – and stop immediately if you feel overexerted. As much as you want to stay in shape, you may have to forgo all exercise until after your babies are safely delivered.

Is it true I'll put on a lot more weight with twins or triplets?

You are more likely to put on extra weight with multiple fetuses. For a normal weight woman, a weight gain of 25–40lb (11–18kg) for a twin birth is recommended. However, some women do not gain as much weight because of the added stress on their bodies.

Is it true that a woman expecting more than one baby has more heartburn than other pregnant women?

This is often the case. It is caused by the larger uterus encroaching on the space the stomach usually enjoys by itself.

I've heard that most complications in a multiple pregnancy arise in the last trimester. Is this true?

Yes, this is true. As the babies grow larger, the mother-to-be may experience more problems. The biggest problem with twins is premature labour and premature delivery. When you are carrying twins, you get 'big' earlier and you get larger than with a single pregnancy. This can cause problems earlier, such as difficulty breathing, back pain, haemorrhoids, varicose veins, pelvic pressure and pelvic pain.

I heard a mother of twins talking at my doctor's surgery. She said she waited too long to buy the things she needed for her babies. What did she mean?

Many expectant mothers wait until they are close to the delivery date of their baby to buy nursery items they will need. However, the expectant mother of twins, triplets and more shouldn't wait this long

– your second trimester is not too early to buy the things you will need. It may be better to choose these things while you can get around easily than to have to wait until after your babies are born!

A friend who had twins told me her doctor advised her to begin her maternity leave from work early. Is this true?
Often a doctor will advise a woman expecting twins to stop working at least 8 weeks before her due date. Ideally, a woman should stop working at 28 weeks with a twin pregnancy or 24 weeks if her job requires standing or physical exertion.

My husband and I want to take childbirth education classes. Can we when we're expecting twins?
It's a very good idea to take these classes for any pregnancy, even twins, triplets or more. However, be realistic and schedule your classes to begin at least *3 months* before your due date. If you have time, a brief course on caesarean section might also be worthwhile if you can find one in your area.

I've heard that multiple pregnancies are usually delivered early. What is the average length of pregnancy with more than one baby?
We try to delay delivery of twins until about 37 weeks of pregnancy, and triplets until about 35 weeks.

How are multiple fetuses usually delivered?
This is somewhat controversial and often depends on how the babies are lying in the uterus. All possible combinations of fetal positions can occur. Some doctors believe two or more babies should always be delivered by caesarean section. When twins are both head first, a vaginal delivery may be attempted. One baby may be delivered vaginally, with the second requiring a caesarean section if it turns, if the cord comes out first or if the second baby is distressed after the first baby is born.

I'm expecting twins, and I want to breast feed. Can I?
Yes, you can. It may be more difficult and more demanding, but many women successfully breast feed twins.

I've heard breast milk and breast feeding are good for twins. Why?
We know that breast milk is especially valuable for small or premature infants; often twins are both. For this reason, if you want to breast feed, go ahead and try it.

We're going to have triplets. Is it possible to breast feed triplets?

If you're going to try to breast feed triplets, you'll find it will be more challenging than breast feeding twins. But it's important to try, if you really want to. One way you may be able to do it is to let each baby breast feed for a bit at a feeding, then supplement with formula. You can also express your milk, and divide it between the three of them. Because triplets are usually small and premature, your breast milk is very valuable to them.

I have a friend who had triplets born 10 weeks early. Her breast milk never came in. Is this common?

No, this is not common. Usually a mother produces breast milk without complications.

What kind of family support would you recommend when my twins are born?

Your time of greatest need will be immediately after your babies are born. Ask for help from family, neighbours and friends for the first 4–6 weeks after you bring your babies home. You may be fairly exhausted yourself, so it's very helpful to have extra pairs of hands available until you all settle into a routine.

I've heard there are some special groups for families with twins, triplets or more. What are they?

There are some wonderful resource groups for parents and families of multiples. Contact them for information and assistance. See the Useful Addresses section at the end of the book.

CHAPTER 8

Changes in your Growing Baby

I'm confused about how my doctor determines when my baby is due. Can you explain it so I can understand it?
Most women don't know the exact date their baby was conceived, but they usually know the day their last menstrual period began. Because ovulation occurs near the middle of their cycle, or about 2 weeks before the beginning of their next period, the doctor uses the date of the last period and adds 2 weeks as an estimate of when conception occurred. Your estimated due date is 38 weeks after the date of conception, or 40 weeks after the last period.

Is there any other way to determine when my baby is due?
Yes. Add 7 days to the date of the beginning of your last menstrual period, then subtract 3 months. This gives you the *approximate* date of delivery. For example, if your last period began on 20 January, your estimated due date is 27 October.

I've heard my doctor talk about the 'gestational age' of my growing baby. What is it?
Gestational age, also called *menstrual age*, dates a pregnancy from the first day of the last menstrual period. It is two weeks longer than the fertilisation age.

Then what is 'fertilisation age' that I heard my doctor's nurse mention?
Fertilisation age, also called *ovulatory age*, is 2 weeks shorter than gestational age and dates from the *actual date of conception*. This is the actual age of the fetus.

Fetus

Yolk sac

The fetus at 6 weeks looks more like a tadpole than a baby.

These dating techniques are confusing. When my doctor says I'm 12 weeks pregnant, how old is my baby?

Most doctors count the time during pregnancy in weeks. If your doctor says you're 12 weeks pregnant, he's referring to the *gestational age.* Your last menstrual period began 12 weeks ago, but you actually conceived *10 weeks ago,* so the fetus is *10 weeks old.*

What is the difference between an embryo and a fetus?

The distinction between 'embryo' and 'fetus' is somewhat arbitrary. During the first 8 weeks of development (10 weeks of gestation), the developing baby is often called an *embryo.* From 8 weeks of development until delivery it is called a *fetus.*

I know my developing baby is going through lots of changes. Can you explain some of them to me?

Your baby grows and changes a great deal during your pregnancy, from a small group of cells to a fully developed baby ready to begin life. Changes are more easily discussed if we look at them in each trimester.

What is a trimester?
The length of your pregnancy is divided into three trimesters, each about 13 weeks long.

How does my baby change during the first trimester?
This trimester is the one of greatest change for any developing fetus. In the first 13 weeks of development, your baby grows from a collection of cells the size of the head of a pin to a fetus the size of a tennis ball. Organs begin developing, and your baby begins to look more normal.

How does my baby change during the second trimester?
At the beginning of the second trimester (14 weeks), your baby weighs less than 1oz (30g) and is only about 4in (10cm) long. By the end of this trimester, he or she is almost 9in (22cm) long and weighs close to 1½lb (0.7kg).

How does my baby change during the third trimester?
Your baby weighs about 1½lb (0.7kg) at the beginning of this trimester (27 weeks) and its crown-to-rump length is under 9in (22cm). When it is delivered, your baby will weigh close to 7½lb (3.4kg) and be about 21in (53cm) long.

I read recently that the baby doesn't change very much after about the 12th week of pregnancy. What does this mean?
Very few, if any, structures in the fetus are formed after the 12th week of your pregnancy. This means your baby forms all of its major organ systems by the end of the first trimester. However, these structures continue to grow and to develop until your baby is born.

What is a full term infant?
A fetus born between 38th and 42nd weeks of pregnancy, it is called a *term* or a *full term baby*.

What is a preterm baby?
If a baby is born before 38 weeks of pregnancy, it is called a *preterm baby*.

What is a post term baby?
A baby delivered at 42 weeks or more of pregnancy is called a *post term baby*.

How big are most babies when they are born?
The weight varies greatly from baby to baby. However the average weight of a baby at term is 7–7$\frac{1}{2}$lb (3.3–3.4kg).

Is there any way to estimate from my size how big my baby will be?
It's very hard to estimate the weight of any baby before birth. Many doctors will take a guess and give a range of a couple of pounds. Some of my estimates have really been off! It's not uncommon to estimate a baby will weigh 8$\frac{1}{2}$lb (3.8kg) and find it's only a 7lb (3.15kg) baby when it's born.

My doctor said that ultrasound scanning can sometimes be used to gauge a baby's weight. Is that true?
Ultrasound scanning is sometimes used to estimate fetal weight, but errors do occur. However, the accuracy of predicting fetal weight with ultrasound is improving.

How does an ultrasound scan measure a baby's weight?
A formula has been established to help estimate fetal weight with ultrasound. Several measurements are used, including the diameter of the baby's head, circumference of the baby's abdomen and length of the femur (thigh-bone) of the baby's leg. Occasionally other fetal measurements are taken.

How accurate is an ultrasound scan in measuring a baby's weight before birth?
It is the test of choice to estimate fetal weight. However, estimates may vary as much as $\frac{1}{2}$lb (225g) in either direction.

I'm 13 weeks pregnant and read that my baby's head is about half or 50 per cent of its body length. Can this be true?
Yes, at this point the head is about half the crown-to-rump length. In 2 months, when you are 21 weeks pregnant, the head will be about one-third of the fetal body. At birth, your baby's head will be one-quarter the size of its body.

My doctor told me that my baby's heart starts beating very early. When does this happen?
By 6 weeks of pregnancy (age of fetus is 4 weeks), the heart tubes fuse and contractions of the heart begin. This can be seen on ultrasound scanning.

Early ultrasound scan done at 6 weeks.

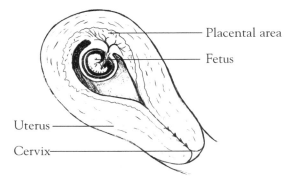

Illustration of what an ultrasound scan shows at 6 weeks.

When will I be able to hear my baby's heart beat?

It may be possible to hear your baby's heart beat with a stethoscope at around 20 weeks of pregnancy. If you can't hear your baby's heart beat with the stethoscope, don't worry. It's not always easy, even for a doctor who does this on a regular basis. With doppler ultrasound, it is possible to hear the heartbeat as early as 12 weeks.

While I was listening to my baby's heart beat the other day at my doctor's surgery, I heard it skip a beat. Is this serious?

An irregular heartbeat is called an *arrhythmia*. Arrhythmias in a fetus are not unusual, so don't be overly concerned about it. Also, the equipment could be faulty or there may be come other problem with transmitting the sound. Your doctor will be on the watch for these kinds of problem; if he or she believes there is a problem with the baby, you may be referred to a perinatologist for further evaluation.

If my baby does have an arrhythmia, what can be done about it?

Arrhythmias are not usually serious in a baby before birth; many disappear after the baby is born. If an arrhythmia is discovered before labour and delivery, you may require fetal heart rate monitoring during pregnancy. When an arrhythmia is discovered during labour, it may be desirable to have a paediatrician present when the baby is born.

How is it decided whether I will have a boy or a girl? Is it very complicated?

The sex of the baby is determined at the time of fertilisation. If a sperm carrying a Y chromosome fertilises the egg, it results in a male child; a sperm carrying an X chromosome results in a female child. It's all determined at the time the sperm fertilises your egg.

When I had my ultrasound scan last week it looked as if my baby had its mouth open. Is that possible?

Yes, it is. In addition to opening and closing its mouth, the fetus may also suck its thumb or finger.

I've heard a developing baby swallows amniotic fluid. Is that true?

By 21 weeks, the fetal digestive system has developed enough to allow the fetus to swallow amniotic fluid. The fetus absorbs much of the water in the swallowed fluid. Hydrochloric acid and adult digestive enzymes are present in small amounts in the fetal digestive system at 21 weeks.

Why does my baby swallow the amniotic fluid?

Researchers believe swallowing amniotic fluid may help growth and development of the fetal digestive system. It may also condition the digestive system to function after birth.

How much fluid does my baby swallow?

By the time a baby is born, he or she may swallow large amounts of amniotic fluid, as much as 17oz (500ml) in 24 hours. This is absorbed and passed into the mother's circulation through the placenta and through the fetal kidneys back into the amniotic cavity.

Does my baby open its eyes inside my uterus?
Eyelids cover the eyes and are fused or connected around 11–12 weeks.
They remain fused until about 27–28 weeks, when they open.

A friend told me a baby can hear inside the womb, before it's born. Is this true?
Yes. Life inside the womb may be like living near a busy airport. The developing baby hears a constant background of digestive noises and the maternal heartbeat. The mother-to-be's voice is also heard, although the fetus may not hear higher pitched tones.

Does my growing baby respond to sounds?
There is evidence that by the third trimester the fetus responds to sounds it hears. Researchers have noted fetal heart rate increases in response to tones it hears through the mother's abdomen.

Will my baby know my voice after he or she is born?
Newborn babies have been found to prefer their mother's voice to a stranger's, which suggests they recognise the mother's voice. They have also been found to prefer their mother's native language, and they respond strongly to a recording of an intra-uterine heartbeat.

Problems for the Developing Fetus

An article I read said early pregnancy is the time the fetus is most susceptible to malformations. What did it mean?
The first 10 weeks of pregnancy (8 weeks of fetal development) are called the *embryonic period*. This is a time of extremely important development in the baby, and the embryo is *most susceptible* to factors that can interfere with its development. Most malformations originate during this period.

What is the chance of my baby having a major birth defect?
Every pregnant couple worries about birth defects. The risk of a major birth defect is 1–2 per cent.

I was reading a book that mentioned 'teratology'. What is that?
Teratology is the study of abnormal fetal development. When a birth defect occurs, we want to know why it happened. This can be frustrating because in most instances we are unable to determine a

cause. A substance that causes birth defects is called a *teratogen* or is said to be *teratogenic*. Some things may have a bad effect (be teratogenic) at one point in pregnancy, then be safe at others.

The most critical time appears to be early in pregnancy, during the first trimester or first 13 weeks. An example of this is rubella (German measles). If the fetus is infected during the first trimester, abnormalities such as heart defects can occur. If infection happens later, problems may be less serious.

Do all the medicines I take affect my baby? I thought some were safe.

Medicines can be grouped into three main groups – safe, unsafe and unsure. It's best to avoid medicines during pregnancy unless you discuss them with your doctor. Some medicines such as thyroid treatment, are necessary and important during pregnancy.

It's easier and safer to discuss this with your doctor beforehand rather than after you have taken the medicine and want to know if it is safe or if it has harmed your baby. For a chart on how some medicines can affect the developing fetus, see page 75.

I read about a baby born with cataracts. I thought that only happened to older people – is it possible?

Congenital (present at birth) cataracts rarely happen and are usually genetic. With cataracts, the lens of the eye is not transparent. Children born to mothers who had German measles (rubella) around the 6th or 7th week of pregnancy may be born with cataracts.

What is microphthalmia?

Microphthalmia is an abnormal congenital condition of the eye in which the overall size of the eyeball is too small. This occurs more often with other problems of the eyes. The cause is generally thought to be infections, such as cytomegalovirus (CMV) or toxoplasmosis.

We live in an area with lots of air pollution. Can my exposure to smog and bad air affect my baby?

This is very rarely a problem and would be very hard to prove. Your lungs and airways filter the air you breathe, and that protects your baby.

Premature Birth

I'm 25 weeks pregnant. If my baby was born now, would it be OK?
It is hard to believe, but some babies born at 25 weeks survive. Some of the greatest advances in medicine have been in the care of premature babies. However, don't start wishing for delivery now; babies born this early are in the hospital a long time and often have serious problems.

Why is it risky for the baby to be born early?
Premature birth increases the risk of physical and/or mental impairment in the baby. It also increases the risk of neonatal death.

How early is 'too early'?
It depends on your particular situation. In many cases, 1 or 2 weeks is not going to make such difference in your baby – the baby may only be slightly smaller. However, the earlier the baby is born, the greater the risks.

I've heard that more premature babies are surviving today. Is that true?
Yes, it is. Because of advances in technology, today fewer than 10 deaths per 1,000 are reported in premature births.

Is it true that premature babies have long hospital stays?
In general, premature babies born after 35 weeks or weighing more than 5.5llbs (2500g) do not need to stay in a hospital for any extra time. However, small premature babies, born before 32 weeks, may have to stay in hospital for 30–100 days.

How are these premature babies affected?
In babies born extremely early, there is an increased rate of physical and mental handicaps, some of them severe. This is the reason your doctor will attempt to prolong your pregnancy as much as possible.

Hydrocephalus

I read an article that talked about hydrocephalus. What is it?
Hydrocephalus is a problem with the development of the baby that causes an enlargement of the head. It occurs in about 1 in 2,000 babies

and is responsible for about 12 per cent of all severe fetal malformations found at birth.

How does hydrocephalus happen?
The organisation and development of the brain and central nervous system of the baby begin early. Cerebro-spinal fluid circulates around the brain and spinal cord, and must be able to flow without restriction. If openings are blocked and the flow of fluid is restricted, it can cause hydrocephalus (sometimes called *water on the brain*). The fluid accumulates and causes the baby's head to enlarge.

If my baby has hydrocephalus, can anything be done?
Hydrocephalus is a symptom and can have several causes, including spina bifida, meningomyelocoele and omphalocoele. Sometimes intra-uterine treatment – while the fetus is still in the uterus – can be performed.

How is hydrocephalus treated inside the uterus?
There are two ways of treating hydrocephalus in utero (inside the uterus). In one method, a needle is passed through the mother's abdomen into the affected area of the baby's brain to remove fluid. In the other method, a small plastic tube is placed into the area of fluid in the fetal brain. This tube is left in place to drain fluid continuously from the baby's brain.

The Presence of Meconium

A couple of friends of mine who've had babies were discussing meconium. What is it?
The term *meconium* refers to undigested debris from swallowed amniotic fluid in the fetal digestive system. It is a greenish-black to light-brown substance that your baby may pass from its bowels into the amniotic fluid. This may happen before or at the time of delivery.

Is meconium important?
The presence of meconium can be important at the time of delivery. If a baby has a bowel movement and meconium is in the amniotic fluid, the infant may swallow the fluid before birth or at the time of birth. If meconium is inhaled into the lungs, it may cause pneumonia or pneumonitis.

Is there any way to know about meconium ahead of time?
Meconium is detected when your water breaks. Before this time, the only way to know about it is by amniocentesis.

If there is meconium present when I am in labour, what can be done?
If meconium is present at the time of delivery, an attempt is made to remove it from the baby's mouth and throat with a small suction tube so the baby won't swallow it.

What causes meconium in the amniotic fluid?
Passage of meconium into the amniotic fluid may be caused by distress in the fetus. When meconium is present, it doesn't always mean distress, but it must be considered.

Intra-uterine Growth Retardation

A friend of mine was telling me her doctor was concerned about intra-uterine growth retardation. It sounds very serious; what is it?
Intra-uterine growth retardation (IUGR) means a newborn baby is small for its age. By medical definition, the baby's weight is in the bottom 10 per cent for the baby's gestational age. This means that 9 out of 10 babies of the same gestational age are larger. The condition is also called *fetal growth retardation*.

If my baby has IUGR, does it mean he or she will be mentally retarded?
No, not usually. The word 'retardation' may cause a mother-to-be some concern. Retardation in this sense does not apply to the development or function of the baby's brain. It does not mean the baby will be mentally retarded. It means the growth and size of the fetus are inappropriately small; *growth* and *size* are considered to be retarded or slowed.

Why is IUGR serious?
When the baby's weight is low, the risk of fetal death increases significantly.

What causes intra-uterine growth retardation?
There are many conditions that increase the chance of IUGR. These include the following situations:

- small size of mother-to-be (probably not a cause for alarm)
- maternal anaemia
- smoking by the mother-to-be during pregnancy
- poor weight gain by the mother-to-be
- vascular disease in the mother-to-be, including high blood pressure
- kidney disease in the mother-to-be
- alcoholism or drug abuse by the pregnant woman
- multiple fetuses
- infections in the fetus
- abnormalities in the umbilical cord or the placenta

If a woman has one baby with IUGR, will her next baby be affected?
Research has shown that a previous delivery of a growth-retarded baby indicates it might happen again in subsequent pregnancies.

How will my doctor know if my baby is too small?
The problem is usually found by watching the growth of your uterus for a period of time and finding no change. If you measure 10.8in (27.4cm) at 27 weeks of pregnancy and at 31 weeks you measure only 11in (28cm), your doctor might become concerned about IUGR. This is one of the important reasons for you to keep all your antenatal appointments.

If IUGR is diagnosed, can anything be done for the baby?
Your doctor will advise you to avoid anything that can make it worse. Stop smoking. Stop using drugs or alcohol. Eat nutritiously. Bed rest may also be prescribed. This allows your baby to receive the best blood flow from you and thus to receive as much nutrition as possible.

What is the most serious risk to a baby with IUGR?
The greatest risk is stillbirth (death of the baby before delivery). It may be necessary to deliver the baby before full term to avoid this.

If I have a baby with IUGR, is it more likely I will have a caesarean section?
Because babies with IUGR may not tolerate labour well, the possibility of a caesarean section increases due to fetal distress. When there is some problem, the baby may be safer outside the uterus than inside.

Umbilical Cord Problems

I heard about a baby born recently that had knots in its umbilical cord. What causes this?
We believe knots in the umbilical cord form as the baby moves around early in pregnancy. A loop forms in the umbilical cord, and when the baby moves through the loop, a knot forms.

I've heard that the baby can get tangled up in the umbilical cord. Is this true?
In some cases this is true, but it usually isn't a problem. There is nothing you can do to prevent this from happening.

Could a tangled cord hurt my baby?
It isn't necessarily a problem. It only becomes a problem if the cord is stretched tightly around the neck or in a tight knot.

Is there anything I can do to keep my baby from getting a knot in its umbilical cord?
No, there is nothing you can do to prevent it. Be reassured that these knots do not occur often.

CHAPTER 9

Changes in You

I know the baby grows and changes a great deal during pregnancy. What can I expect for me?
The time of pregnancy is an exciting time for you and may be a little frightening, too. You will see yourself change in many ways – your abdomen will grow much larger, your breasts will enlarge, you may experience some swelling in the hands and feet, and you may experience many other changes. By being aware of these changes, you should be more comfortable with them.

What changes will I see during the first trimester?
You will see very little change in yourself, although your baby is growing and changing quite rapidly. You may not even realise you are pregnant until the middle or close to the end of this trimester! You will experience very little weight gain during this time – probably no more than 5lb (2.25kg) for the entire 13 weeks. Your abdomen will grow a little – you may be able to feel your uterus about 3in (7.6cm) below your belly button. You won't feel the fetus move during this time.

What changes will I see during the second trimester?
You will begin showing to others you are pregnant during this trimester. You will be able to feel your uterus about 3in (7.6cm) *below* your belly button at the beginning of this trimester. By the end, you will feel your uterus about 3in (7.6cm) *above* your belly button.

Average weight gain for this trimester is a total (including weight from the first trimester) of 14–20lb (6–9kg). You will begin to feel your baby move during this time.

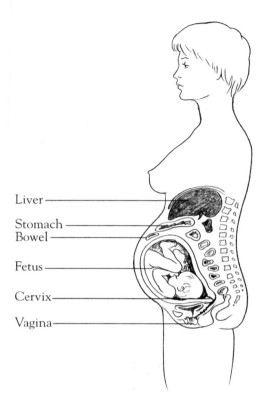

Liver

Stomach

Bowel

Fetus

Cervix

Vagina

*A pregnant woman's uterus takes up a great deal of space in the abdominal cavity.
Other organs are pushed out of the way, which can make the woman feel very
uncomfortable.*

What changes will I see during the third trimester?

You will experience a great deal of change in you during this time
because your baby will be growing so much. You will be able to feel
your uterus about 3in (7.6cm) above your belly button at the
beginning of this trimester. By delivery, you will feel your uterus
6¹/₂–8in (16.5–20.3cm) above your belly button.

Your baby will be gaining a great deal of weight during this time,
even though you may not. Total weight gain by delivery is 18–28lb
(8–13kg) for the average woman.

What can I do about the changes I go through during pregnancy?
The most important thing you can do for yourself is to get good antenatal care. Follow your doctor's recommendations about nutrition, medication and exercise. Keep all your appointments. Establish good communication with your doctor or midwife. Ask any question that bothers you.

My cousin said that with her second and third pregnancies her body started to change much earlier than with her first pregnancy. Why?
The way a woman's body responds to pregnancy is influenced by her previous pregnancies. Skin and muscles stretch to accommodate the enlarged uterus, placenta and baby. Stretched muscles and stretched skin are never exactly the same again. They may give way faster to

38 weeks
30 weeks
26 weeks
18 weeks
8 weeks

This illustration shows how a woman's uterus grows during pregnancy. The dotted lines represent growth from about 8 weeks to the end of the third trimester (about 38 weeks).

accommodate the growing uterus and baby with subsequent pregnancies, which causes a woman to show sooner and feel bigger.

I'm 11 weeks pregnant and know I'm almost done with the first trimester, but I don't even show yet. Should I be concerned?
No. A lot has been happening with the development of your baby's organs and organ systems. However, friends are probably not yet able to tell you're pregnant. You may be able to feel your uterus down by your pubic bone or your clothes may be getting a little snug.

If this is your first pregnancy, it often takes longer to see a change in your 'tummy'. If you have had other pregnancies, you will probably show sooner. Don't despair – you'll be getting larger soon, then everyone will know you're pregnant!

I'm not very far along and feel a lot bigger than with my last pregnancy. Is this all right?
It isn't unusual to show sooner or feel bigger if you have had other pregnancies. You can blame the other pregnancies for stretching your skin and muscles so that you show sooner. It is also possible that you are farther along than you think or you are carrying twins! Discuss it with your doctor if you are concerned.

Everyone tells me I'm too big. What's wrong?
Before you become overly concerned, discuss it with your doctor or midwife. Friends may tell you you are too big or too small; probably nothing is wrong. Women and babies are different sizes and grow at different rates. What is of greatest importance is the continual change and continual growth of the fetus.

Changes in your Skin

I've noticed a dark line has appeared on my abdomen. What is it?
The vertical line that appears down the midline of your abdomen is called the *linea nigra*. It appears on many women during pregnancy.

Will this line disappear after pregnancy?
The linea nigra often fades markedly after pregnancy, but it may never fully disappear.

I've got brown patches on my face that I never had before. What are they?

Occasionally irregular brown patches appear on the face and neck of a pregnant woman. Patches are called *chloasma* or *mask of pregnancy* and are believed to be caused by the hormone changes brought about during pregnancy. Usually these dark patches disappear completely or get lighter after your baby is born. (Oral contraceptives often cause similar pigmentation changes.)

Since I became pregnant, I've noticed some small red elevations on the skin of my neck and upper chest. What causes this?

During pregnancy, you may experience vascular changes to your skin. These small red elevations, with branches extending outwards, are called *spider naevi*, *telangiectasias* or *angiomas*. They usually occur on the face, neck, upper chest and arms, and will disappear after delivery.

My sister-in-law had red palms all during her pregnancy. is this common?

The condition you're referring to, called *palmar erythema*, is not uncommon. It occurs in 65 per cent of pregnant white women and 35 per cent of pregnant black women. It is probably caused by increased oestrogen in the system and is usually symptomless. It's all right to use lotions but the redness of your palms may not disappear until after you deliver.

Can spider naevi and red palms occur together?

Yes, they often occur together. Symptoms are temporary and disappear shortly after delivery. Researchers believe the occurrence of these conditions is caused by high levels of oestrogen during pregnancy.

I've noticed that I have a mole that seems to be getting larger. Is this something I should be concerned about?

Pregnancy can cause many changes in your skin. Moles may appear for the first time, or existing moles may grow larger and darken during pregnancy. If you have a mole that changes, be sure to have your doctor check it.

I have little tags of skin that seemed to have grown since I became pregnant. What are they?

Skin tags are small lumps or bumps of skin that may appear for the first time during pregnancy. If you already have them, they may grow larger while you are pregnant. Don't worry too much about them. If they are in an area that is rubbed frequently, you may want to talk to your doctor about removing them.

I've noticed since I've been pregnant that my skin feels itchy, and I scratch a lot. Does this indicate a problem?

Itching, also called *pruritis gravidarum*, is a common symptom during pregnancy. It usually occurs later in pregnancy, and about 20 per cent of all pregnant women suffer from it. Itching does not indicate any problem in your pregnancy.

The skin over my abdomen itches the most. What causes this?

As your uterus grows and fills your pelvis, abdominal skin and muscles must stretch to accommodate it. Stretching of the skin causes abdominal itching in many women.

What can I do about this itching?

If you scratch the skin, it can make it worse, so try not to scratch. These are lotions available to help reduce the itching. Occasionally cortisone creams are used. Ask your doctor about relief.

I've noticed I've had flareups of spots lately. Is this related to my pregnancy?

Most women experience some changes in their skin while pregnant. Some women find their skin breaks out more often. Some lucky women find their skin becomes less oily and softer. These changes are due to the hormones of pregnancy; your skin will probably return to normal after your baby is born.

My dermatologist has just told me I have a couple of precancerous spots on my face. I've had then before and usually get them removed. Can I do this during pregnancy, or should I wait until after the baby is born?

Yes, you can have these spots removed. This is usually done in the doctor's surgery and is not a problem.

What are stretch marks?

Stretch marks, also called *striae gravidarum*, are areas of stretched skin that may be discoloured. They usually occur on the abdomen as your growing uterus stretches the skin. They can also occur on the breasts, hips or buttocks.

Will my stretch marks go away after my pregnancy?
Stretch marks usually fade and won't be as noticeable after your pregnancy, but they won't go away completely.

Is there anything I can do to avoid getting stretch marks?
No one has found a reliable way of avoiding stretch marks. Women have tried many kinds of lotions with little success. There is no harm in trying olive oil or lotions, but they probably won't help.

Varicose Veins

My mother had varicose veins during her pregnancies. Will I?
Varicose veins, also called *varicosities* or *varices*, occur to some degree in most pregnant women. There seems to be an inherited predisposition to varicose veins that can become more severe during pregnancy. If your mother had varicose veins, you have a greater chance of having them.

What causes varicose veins?
Varicose veins (varices) are dilated blood vessels that fill up with blood. They usually occur in the legs but also may be seen as haemorrhoids or appear in the birth canal and in the vulva. The pressure from the uterus and the change in blood flow make varices worse.

What do varicose veins look like?
Symptoms vary. For some women varicose veins are only a blemish or purple-blue spot on the legs. These cause little or no discomfort, except in the evening. For other women, varices are bulging veins that require elevation of the legs at the end of the day.

Will varicose veins get worse during pregnancy?
They may. In most cases, they become more noticeable and more painful as pregnancy progresses. Increasing weight (from your growing baby), clothing that constricts at the waist or legs, and standing a great deal will cause them to worsen.

If I have varicose veins, what can I do?
Many women wear maternity support tights; there are various types available. Clothes that don't restrict circulation at the knee or groin may also help. Spend as little time as possible on your feet. Elevate

your feet above the level of your heart or lie on your side when possible to allow drainage of the veins. Wear flat shoes. Don't cross your legs when you sit down. It you continue to have problems after your pregnancy, surgery may be required.

Friends who have varicose veins say the maternity support tights really do work, but they are almost impossible to put on. Do you have any suggestions?
Support tights can be very different to put on, but there are a couple of tricks that can help you get them on more easily. First, turn tights inside out. Starting at the toe, unroll the tights up your legs. Second, put your support tights on *before* you get out of bed in the morning – your legs may tend to swell as soon as you get up.

Is there anything I can do during pregnancy to decrease my chances of getting varicose veins?
There are some things you can do to help decrease your chances of developing varicose veins. Some of these practices are the same ones you would use if you already suffer from varicose veins.

- Exercise.
- Don't cross your legs at the knee.
- Don't stand for long periods of time.
- If you must stand, bounce gently on the balls of your feet every few minutes.
- Elevate your legs above the level of your heart or lie on your side several times a day.
- Keep your total pregnancy weight gain in the normal range – 24–28lb (11–13kg) for a normal weight woman.

Emotional Changes during Pregnancy

I seem to cry at the least little thing. Why does this happen?
Crying easily, mood swings, energy lows and fatigue are all normal aspects of pregnancy. During the first trimester of pregnancy, your body experiences an increase in hormones that are needed to support a pregnancy. Some women are more sensitive to these changes, especially those who are sensitive to a similar hormone shift before menstruation. If you become weepy or edgy around your menstrual period, you may experience similar emotions as your body adjusts to pregnancy.

I am experiencing conflicting feelings about my pregnancy. Is this normal?
It is very normal. Your conflicting feelings arise from your adjustment to your pregnancy – you are taking the first steps towards an incredible role change that will involve many aspects of your life. Your feelings of conflict come from your attempts to deal with all the questions and concerns you have.

I've been very depressed during my pregnancy. Should I ask my doctor for an anti-depressant?
Anti-depressant medicines are not usually prescribed during pregnancy because they are not considered safe at this time. However, if it is necessary, most doctors prefer to use tricyclic anti-depressants, such as amitriptyline and desipramine. Treatment must be done on an individualised basis. Your doctor and possibly a psychiatrist or psychologist will discuss the situation with you.

I'm in my third trimester and seem to be more emotional than ever. Is there anything wrong me me?
No, you're normal. You may be getting a little more anxious about the approaching labour and delivery. You may find mood swings occur more frequently, and you may be more irritable. Try to relax and not focus on your feelings. Talk to your partner about how you are feeling and what you are experiencing.

Some Discomforts of Pregnancy

I have terrible morning sickness. When will it end?
By the end of the first trimester, most women experience an improvement in morning sickness. For more information on this, see Chapter 2.

Is it true that it's not unusual to experience pain in the uterus during pregnancy?
As your uterus grows during pregnancy, you may feel slight cramping or even pain in your lower abdominal area and in your sides. Your uterus will tighten or contract throughout your pregnancy. If you don't feel this, don't worry. However, if contractions are accompanied by bleeding from the vagina, call your doctor immediately!

A friend mentioned Braxton-Hicks contractions. What are they?

Braxton-Hicks contractions during pregnancy are painless, non-rhythmical contractions you may be able to feel when you place your hands on your abdomen. You may also feel them in the uterus itself. These contractions may being early in your pregnancy and are felt at irregular intervals. They are not signs of true labour.

I've had a weird feeling in my pelvic area – sort of a 'pins and needles' feeling. Is there something wrong?

Not usually. This is another feeling associated with increased pressure as the baby moves lower in the birth canal. Tingling, pressure and numbness are common at this time and shouldn't concern you.

Can I do anything to alleviate any of this pressure?

Lie on your side to help decrease pressure in your pelvis and on the nerves, veins and arteries in your pelvic area.

When I move or get up, my sides hurt. Should I worry?

Probably not. What you are describing is usually called *round ligament pain*. The round ligaments are on either side of the uterus; as your uterus gets bigger, these ligaments stretch and get longer and thicker. Quick movements can stretch these ligaments and hurt. This is not harmful to you or your baby, but it can be uncomfortable.

What can I do for round ligament pain?

Be careful about making sudden movements. It may feel better to lie down and rest. Most doctors recommend paracetamol (Panadol) if the pain bothers you. Tell your doctor if it gets worse.

Feeling your Baby Move

My friend was talking about 'quickening'. What is it?

Quickening is feeling your baby move. It usually occurs between 16 and 20 weeks of pregnancy.

I'm 15 weeks pregnant and have already felt my baby move. Is there something wrong?

The time at which you first feel your baby move is different for every woman. It can also be different from one pregnancy to another. One baby may be more active than another, so movement is felt sooner.

I thought I felt my baby move when I was 11 weeks pregnant, but my doctor said it was probably wind. How will I know that what I feel is my baby moving?

Many women describe the first feelings of movement from their baby as a gas bubble or fluttering in their abdomen. It may be something you notice for a few days before you realise what it is. Movements will be more common and occur fairly frequently – that's how you'll know that what you're feeling is your baby moving. The movement will be below your belly button. If it's your first baby, it may be 19 or 20 weeks before you are sure you feel movement.

I'm in the early part of my second trimester, and I haven't felt my baby move yet. Is that all right?

Yes. The normal time to feel movement is between 16 and 20 weeks.

I felt my baby move for the first time last week but haven't felt it for a couple of days. What's wrong?

Probably nothing. It is normal not to feel it every day at first. As your baby grows, you'll feel movements become stronger and probably more regular.

My friend, who is also pregnant, complains that her baby moves all the time. My baby doesn't move that much. Should I be worried?

This is a hard question to answer. Your sensation of your baby moving is different from your friend's, and the movement of every baby is different. It isn't unusual for one baby to move less than another. If your baby has been very active then is very quiet for a while, you may want to discuss it with your doctor. He or she will determine if there is any reason for concern.

My baby is extremely active during the night, and it keeps me awake. Is there anything I can do about it?

There really isn't much you can do about this. You might try changing your position in bed. Avoid exercising just before bed – it may cause your baby to move more. If these tips don't work, you may have to be patient and just endure it until your baby is born.

My baby kicks a lot, and it hurts. Is there anything I can do to make him or her stop?

Try changing your position and lying on one side. It may still be uncomfortable. Taking paracetamol or relaxing in a warm (not hot) bath may also help.

I get a sort of pain under my ribs sometimes when my baby is active. Can I do anything about it?

There isn't very much you can do about the pain or the pressure you feel when your baby moves. You might try lying on your side and resting for a while. For example, if you feel pressure under your right ribs, lie on your left side.

A friend of mine is 26 weeks pregnant. Her doctor wants her to keep track of her baby's movements. Why?

A doctor may have a mother-to-be monitor her baby's movements around this time if she has had a difficult pregnancy, if she had a previous stillbirth or if she has a medical condition, such as diabetes. Recording the movements at certain times each day may provide the doctor with additional information about the baby's progress.

Between 20 and 32 weeks of pregnancy, the fetus can move between 200 and 500 times a day, including kicking, rolling or wiggling.

My doctor said my baby is 'floating'. What did she mean?

This means the baby can be felt at the beginning of the birth canal, but it has not dropped into the birth canal. That is, the baby is not engaged (fixed) in the birth canal at this time. The baby may even move away from your doctor's fingers when you are examined.

I feel as though my baby is going to fall out. This can't happen, can it?

No, it can't. What you are probably experiencing is the pressure of your baby as it moves lower in the birth canal. If this occurs, bring it to your doctor's attention. He or she may want to do a pelvic examination to check how low the baby's head is.

Constipation

I've never had constipation before. Why do I have it now?

It is common during pregnancy for bowel habits to change. Most women notice an increase in constipation, often accompanied by irregular bowel habits and an increase in the occurrence of haemorrhoids. These problems are usually the result of a slowdown in the movement of food through the gastrointestinal system and of iron supplements or iron in antenatal vitamins.

What can I do to relieve constipation?
There are some things you can do to help relieve the problem. Increase your fluid intake, and exercise three or four times a week. Many doctors suggest prune juice or a mild laxative, such as Milk of Magnesia. Certain foods that are high in fibre, such as bran and prunes, increase the bulk in your diet and may help relieve constipation.

Can I take laxatives to relieve the constipation?
Do *not* use laxatives, other than those mentioned above, without consulting your doctor. If your constipation is a continuing problem, discuss it with your doctor.

Taking Care of your Teeth

I've always heard that a woman should avoid any dental treatment when she is pregnant. Is this true?
No! As a matter of fact, you should have regular dental checkups during your pregnancy. They are very important.

My gums seem to be bleeding more now that I'm pregnant. Should I be concerned?
Pregnancy can cause sore, bleeding, swollen gums because of the hormone changes your body goes through. Your gums are more susceptible to irritation and may bleed more often when you floss or brush your teeth.

Will my gums get better after pregnancy?
Yes. The condition usually clears up by itself after the baby is born. Talk to your dentist if the problem becomes too uncomfortable.

Should I tell my dentist I'm pregnant.
Yes. If you need any dental treatment, advise your dentist you are pregnant before anything is done. Some dental anaesthetics might harm your baby. In most cases, a pregnant woman should not have a general anaesthetic.

I have a small nodule on my gum that bleeds when I brush it. What is it?
This is called a *pyogenic granuloma* or *pregnancy tumour* and may bleed when you brush your teeth or eat. This condition usually clears up after pregnancy, but don't ignore it if it causes you problems.

I was due to have cosmetic bonding done to my teeth then found out I was pregnant. Should I cancel my appointment?

I usually advise a pregnant woman to wait until after the baby is born to have any *elective* dental procedure. However, if you have a dental trauma, such as an abscess or a broken tooth, get it taken care of immediately!

I usually have X-rays at my dental checkups. Should I have them now?

Be sure you tell your dentist you are pregnant before he or she begins your examination. In most cases, avoid dental X-rays while you are pregnant. If there is a particular need for them, discuss the problem with your dentist *and* your doctor before proceeding any further. If you *must* have an X-ray, shield your pregnancy with a lead apron.

I had to have a root canal done last year and had to take antibiotics before the procedure. If I have the same kind of problem while I'm pregnant, should I take antibiotics?

You must discuss this situation with both your dentist and your doctor. They will be able to decide the best course of action. You must understand that taking care of this kind of problem is important – an infection in you might possibly harm the baby. Together, your dentist and doctor will plan the safest course of treatment for you and your baby.

Are there any ways I can help keep my teeth in good shape during pregnancy?

There are many things you can do yourself to keep your teeth and gums healthy while you are pregnant. Follow these tips.

- Brush your teeth after every meal.
- Floss teeth at least once a day.
- Have at least one check up and dental cleaning during pregnancy, preferably after the first trimester.
- Watch your diet. Eat foods rich in vitamin C (good for gums) and calcium (to keep teeth healthy).
- If you have morning sickness, rinse teeth thoroughly after vomiting.

Miscellaneous Problems you may Experience

I have just found out I'm 9 weeks pregnant, and I have to go to the bathroom all the time. Does this last all through pregnancy?
One of the first symptoms of early pregnancy is frequent urination. This problem continues off and on throughout pregnancy; you may have to get up to go to the bathroom at night when you never did before. It usually lessens during the second trimester, then returns during the third trimester, when the growing baby puts pressure on the bladder.

My friend, who is also pregnant, told me she has a urinary tract infection. She said it's common in pregnancy. Is it?
It is more common to get urinary tract infections during pregnancy. They are also called *bladder infections, cystitis* and *UTIs*.

How will I know if I have a urinary tract infection?
Symptoms include painful urination, a burning during urination, feeling an urgent wish to urinate, blood in the urine and frequent urination.

Can I do anything to avoid a urinary tract infection?
You can do yourself a favour by not 'holding' your urine. Empty your bladder as soon as you feel you need to. Drink plenty of fluids. Cranberry juice helps acidify your urine (kills bacteria) and may help you avoid infections. For some women, it helps to urinate after having intercourse.

Can a urinary tract infection harm my baby?
A urinary tract infection during pregnancy may be a cause of premature labour and low birth weight infants. If you think you have an infection, discuss it with your doctor. If you do have an infection, take the entire prescription of antibiotics prescribed for you.

Ever since I got pregnant, I've noticed I have more vaginal discharge. Is this a sign of a problem?
No. it's normal to have an increase in vaginal discharge or vaginal secretion during pregnancy. It is called *leucorrhoea*. The discharge is usually white or yellow and fairly thick. It is unlikely to be an infection if it is not itching.

What causes the increase in vaginal secretions?

We believe it is caused by the increased blood flow to the skin and muscles around the vagina, which also causes *Chadwick's sign* in early pregnancy. This symptom is visible to your doctor as a violet or blue coloration of your vagina when he or she does a pelvic examination. (It's one of the reasons your doctor performs a pelvic examination on you in early pregnancy.)

How do I treat this vaginal discharge?

Do *not* douche if you have a heavy vaginal discharge during pregnancy. Wear sanitary pads for protection. Avoid wearing tights and nylon underwear – choose cotton underwear or underwear with a cotton gusset.

What if the vaginal discharge is caused by an infection? How will I know?

The discharge that accompanies a vaginal infection is often foul-smelling, has a greenish or yellowish colour, and causes itching or irritation around or inside the vagina. If you have any of these symptoms, notify your doctor. Treatment is often possible; there are many creams and ointments available that are safe to use during pregnancy.

Changes in your Breasts

I'm 13 weeks pregnant and my breasts are getting bigger. Isn't this a little early?

There are many changes in your breasts during pregnancy. After about 8 weeks, it's normal for your breasts to start getting larger. You may even notice they are lumpy or nodular. These are all normal changes in pregnancy.

My breasts are very tender and sore. Is this normal?

Tenderness, tingling or soreness of your breasts early in pregnancy is common.

I've noticed the area around my nipples is getting darker. Should I be concerned?

No, this is normal. The nipple is surrounded by the *areola*. Before pregnancy the areola is usually pink but turns brown or red-brown and may get larger during pregnancy and lactation (when you are producing milk).

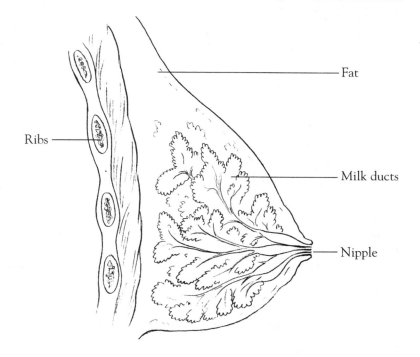

Fat

Ribs

Milk ducts

Nipple

A pregnant woman's breasts change a great deal during pregnancy. One of the greatest changes is the increase in the number of milk ducts which prepare the breast for nursing.

I've noticed some fluid coming from my breasts, staining my clothes. I'm only about halfway through my pregnancy. Is this breast milk already?

No, it isn't. During the second trimester, a thin yellow fluid called *colostrum* is formed; it is the precursor to breast milk. Sometimes it will leak from the breasts or can be expressed by squeezing the nipples. This is normal. It is usually best to leave your breasts alone; don't try to express the fluid. Wear breast pads if you have problems with leakage.

I've heard about 'inverted nipples', but don't know what that means. Can you tell me more about them?

Some women have inverted nipples, which are nipples that are flat or that invert (retract) into the breast. Women with inverted nipples may find it more difficult to breast feed. Ask your doctor about this. There are devices you can use to help prepare your breasts for nursing and make it possible for you to breast feed your baby.

How can I tell if I have inverted nipples?
To determine if you have inverted nipples, place your thumb and index finger on the areola, the dark area surrounding the nipple. Gently compress the base of the nipple. If it flattens or retracts into the breast, you have inverted nipples.

Can I do anything about inverted nipples?
Yes. You can begin wearing breast shells during the last few weeks of pregnancy. These plastic shells are worn under your bra and create a slight pressure at the base of the nipple. This pressure helps draw the nipple out. Ask your doctor or midwife for further information.

I know it sounds silly, but I read in one of the supermarket magazines about a woman who got pregnant, and her breasts went from a size 34B to a size 56H. Is this possible?
Your breasts will enlarge during your pregnancy. However, an increase of this type would be extremely unlikely.

Other Changes you Experience

When will I have to start wearing maternity clothes?
By the beginning of the second trimester (around 14 weeks of pregnancy), maternity clothes will probably be a necessity. If this is your first pregnancy, you may not need maternity clothes until a little later. Also see the discussion of maternity clothes in Chapter 16.

I'm 18 weeks pregnant, and I'm having trouble getting into my clothes. Is it time for me to get maternity clothes?
When your clothes don't fit well and you're uncomfortable, it's time for more comfortable clothes. You still may not 'show' a lot, but it's important to wear clothes that you feel comfortable in. There are many choices for pregnant women, so you should be able to find clothes that are comfortable and support you as you grow bigger.

I've noticed that my hair has been growing faster and feels thicker now that I'm pregnant. Is this common?
Changes in your hair are often triggered by the pregnancy hormones circulating through your body. You may also notice less hair loss than usual. Unfortunately, after your baby is born, the hair you have been retaining during pregnancy is lost. Don't worry about it if it happens to you – you're *not* going bald!

My nails, which have always been soft and hard to grow, are now long and grow very fast. Will they always be like this?
The same hormones that grow your hair also influence your nails. You may find during pregnancy that you have problems keeping your nails filed to a practical length. Enjoy them while you're pregnant. They probably won't last.

I seem to be getting more facial hair now that I'm pregnant. Is this normal?
Some women find they have an increase of facial hair during pregnancy. Usually it's not a problem, but check with your doctor if it worries you. Facial hair will probably disappear or decrease after the pregnancy, so wait before making any decisions about permanent hair removal.

I've been perspiring a lot during my pregnancy. Why?
Pregnancy hormones elevate your body temperature slightly, which may lead to greater perspiration. Use absorbent talc to help keep you dry. If you perspire heavily, make sure you keep you fluid intake up to avoid dehydration.

When I'm lying down and look at my stomach, there's a bulge there I didn't have before (not the baby). Is this the sign of a problem?
Abdominal muscles are stretched and pushed apart as your baby grows. Muscles that are attached to the lower portion of your ribs may separate in the midline, which is called a *diastasis recti*. It isn't painful, and it does not harm the baby.

Will this go away after pregnancy?
It may still be present after the birth of your baby, but the separation won't be as noticeable. Exercising can strengthen the muscles, but you may still have a small bulge or gap.

Every time I go to the doctor, she measures my stomach with a tape measure. Why?
As you progress in your pregnancy, your doctor needs a point of reference to measure how much your uterus is growing. Some measure from the belly button to the top of the uterus. Others measure from the *symphysis pubis*, the place where the pubic bones meet in the middle-lower part of your abdomen, to the top of the uterus.

What kind of things can these measurements tell her?

These measurements can reveal a great deal. If, at 20 weeks, you measure 11.2in (28cm), your doctor may be concerned about the possibility of twins or an incorrect due date. If you measure 6in (15cm) at this point, your due date may be wrong or there may be a concern about intra-uterine growth retardation or some other problem. In either case, your doctor would probably have you further evaluated by ultrasound scanning.

I'm due in about two weeks, and I've noticed a change in the shape of my abdomen – it seems lower. Should I be concerned about this?

Often, a few weeks before labour begins or at the beginning of labour, the head of your baby begins to enter the birth canal and your uterus seems to 'drop' a bit. This is called *lightening*. Don't be concerned if this occurs.

A friend told me that when her baby dropped, she felt better. Why?

One benefit of your baby dropping is an increase in space in your upper abdomen, which gives you more room to breathe. However, as your baby descends, you may notice more pressure in your pelvis, bladder and rectum, which may make you uncomfortable.

Someone told me that my centre of gravity changes during pregnancy. How does this affect me?

When your uterus grows, it grows out in front of you, and the centre of gravity moves forward over your lower extremities (your legs). There is also an increased mobility of your joints. That is, the joints are looser and it may feel as if they are slipping. This can bring about a change in posture, which may cause backache.

I'm 19 weeks pregnant and have only gained 4lb (1.8kg). Should I be concerned?

Weight gain can vary a great deal. If you were sick a lot or had nausea during the first few months, you may have lost weight at first and may be a little behind in gaining weight. If you were overweight before you got pregnant, you may not have gained as much. At this point, you should be gaining weight regularly. Discuss it with your doctor if you are concerned.

CHAPTER 10

Sex during Pregnancy

My husband and I are concerned about sexual activity during pregnancy. What should we do?
Discuss this question with your doctor. You need to rule out any complications and ask for individual advice. Most doctors agree sex can be a part of a normal pregnancy.

My partner is scared to have sex with me because he's afraid it will hurt the baby. What can I tell him?
Sexual activity doesn't usually harm a growing baby. Neither intercourse nor orgasm should be a problem if you have a healthy pregnancy. The baby is well protected by the amniotic sac and amniotic fluid. Uterine muscles are strong and protect the baby, and a thick mucus plug seals the cervix, which helps protect against infection.

Often it's the man who asks about sex during pregnancy. If your partner goes with you to see your doctor, he or you can raise the subject at the next appointment. If he doesn't, assure him there should be no problems if the pregnancy is normal.

After my husband and I have sex, I feel the baby move a lot. Is this because we had sex?
You baby moves a lot, no matter what you are doing. If you feel it move after sexual intercourse, it doesn't mean it was disturbed, uncomfortable or in danger.

My partner and I enjoy sex a lot. Is this bad for me or the baby?
Frequent sexual activity should not be harmful to a healthy pregnancy. Usually a couple can continue the level of sexual activity they are used to. If you are concerned, discuss it with your doctor.

I read that some women have a greater desire for sex during pregnancy. Is this true?

It has been reported by researchers that pregnancy does enhance the sex drive for some women. Some women may experience orgasms or multiple orgasms for the first time during pregnancy. This is due to the heightened hormone activity and increased blood flow to the pelvis.

Physically, I don't feel very much like having sex. Why?

During the first trimester, you may have experienced fatigue and nausea. During the third trimester, your weight gain, your enlarging abdomen, tender breasts and other problems may make you feel less like having sex. This is normal. Tell your partner how you are feeling, and try to work out a solution that is good for both of you.

I don't feel very sexy now that I'm pregnant. Is this normal?

You my feel less attractive now that you're pregnant, but many men find a pregnant woman *very* attractive. If you are experiencing these feelings, discuss them with your partner.

Isn't there some happy medium to my feelings about sex during pregnancy?

According to research, women generally experience one of two sex drive patterns. One is a lessening of desire in the first and third trimesters, with an increase in the second trimester. The second is a gradual decrease in desire for sex as the pregnancy progresses. Sex is individual; you're not going to fit any pattern perfectly. Discuss your feelings with your partner. Tenderness and understanding can help you both.

I feel physically uncomfortable having sex because my body is changing. What can we do about it?

You may find new positions for lovemaking are necessary as your pregnancy progresses. Your larger abdomen may make some positions more uncomfortable than others. In addition, physicians advise a woman not to lie flat on her back from the beginning of the third trimester until the birth. The weight of the uterus restricts circulation. Try lying on your side or with you on top.

What should I do if I have problems or concerns?

As I stated before, discuss any complications and concerns with your doctor throughout your pregnancy. If you have any unusual symptoms during or following sexual activity, discuss them with your doctor *before* resuming sex.

What about sex and miscarriage?
If you have a history of miscarriage, your doctor may caution you against sex and orgasm. However, there is no data that actually links sex and miscarriage.

My friend told me that having sex can cause me to go into labour early. Is this true?
Orgasm causes mild uterine contractions, so if you have a history of early labour your doctor may warn against intercourse and orgasm. Chemicals in semen may also stimulate contractions, so it may not be advisable for the woman's partner to ejaculate inside her. However, in a normal pregnancy, even one near delivery, this is usually not a problem.

What should we avoid during sex now that I'm pregnant?
Some practices should be avoided during sex if you're pregnant. Don't insert any object into the vagina that could cause injury or infection. Blowing air into the vagina is dangerous because it can force a potentially fatal air bubble into the woman's bloodstream. Nipple stimulation releases *oxytocin*, which causes uterine contractions. You might want to discuss this with your doctor.

Are there times we should avoid sex during pregnancy?
Avoid sexual activity if you have any of the following problems or conditions:

- placenta praevia or a low-lying placenta
- incompetent cervix
- premature labour
- multiple fetuses
- ruptured bag of waters
- pain
- unexplained vaginal bleeding or discharge
- you can't find a comfortable position
- either partner has an unhealed herpes lesion
- you believe labour has begun

CHAPTER 11

Your Partner and your Pregnancy

How should I involve my partner before we try to conceive?
Getting pregnant and having a baby involves *both* of you. Talk about the decision to get pregnant, your health and your partner's health. Do this before you try to get pregnant.

How much should my partner be involved in my pregnancy?
Your partner can be a very important source of support for you. It's probably a good idea to involve him as much as he is willing to be involved. Make him feel he's a part of what's going on.

How can I involve my partner more in my pregnancy?
Because the pregnant woman is the focus during pregnancy, a man may feel left out. Educate him so he understands what you and the baby are going through. Share this book and other books and information you receive with him. Take him with you to see the doctor.

My husband seems to find me very sexy now that I'm beginning to show. Is sex all right during pregnancy?
In a normal pregnancy, sex can be a wonderful experience for you both. For a more detailed discussion of sex during pregnancy, see Chapter 10.

My partner isn't as enthusiastic as I am about the approaching birth of our first baby. Is this normal?
Few expectant fathers are as excited about the impending birth as the mother-to-be is. You are directly involved in the pregnancy because you are carrying the baby. Your partner is less involved, so you may have to adjust your expectations somewhat. You may need to take an active role in encouraging your partner to become more involved, such

as asking him to accompany you to an antenatal visit. Discuss with him his feelings about the pregnancy. He may have fears and uncertainties he hasn't voiced to you. Be open and direct with each other about your feelings – it will help both of you.

Is it all right for my husband to go to my antenatal appointments with me?

It's actually a great idea for him to accompany you. It will help him realise what is happening to you and may help him feel more as if he's a part of the pregnancy. It's also good for your husband and your doctor or midwife to meet before labour begins.

My partner seems very anxious about my pregnancy. Is this normal?

Your partner may feel increased anxiety as your pregnancy progresses. He may be concerned about your health, the health of the baby, sex, labour and delivery, and his abilities to be a good father. Share your own concerns with him. It may help calm his anxieties.

My husband wants to know how he can make our pregnancy easier for me. What can I tell him?

A man can help his pregnant partner in many ways.

• Keep stress to a minimum.
• Communicate about everything.
• Be patient and supportive.
• Promote good nutrition.
• Encourage exercise.
• Help around the house when possible, and do the more strenuous chores.
• Attend antenatal check ups when possible.
• Plan for the baby's arrival.
• Learn about the birth process.

I've heard the baby's father can begin bonding with the baby as soon as it is born. How can he do this?

The baby's father can begin bonding with the baby before birth and continue after the baby is born. Encourage your partner to try the following suggestions.

• Have your partner talk to the baby while it is in the uterus.
• Encourage your partner to talk to the baby soon after birth. Babies bond to sound very quickly.

- Have your partner hold the baby close and make eye contact; a baby relates to people through sight and smell.
- Let your partner feed the baby. It's easy if you bottle feed.
- If you breast feed, let him give the baby a bottle of your expressed breast milk.
- Encourage him to help with daily chores, such as changing nappies, holding the baby when it is restless, dressing and bathing the baby.

This may sound weird, but I've head that a man can suffer from morning sickness when his wife is pregnant. Is this true?
Many a father-to-be experiences some sort of physical problem during his wife's pregnancy. The condition is called *couvade*, and originated in a Carib Indian tribe in which every expectant father engages in rituals that enable him to understand what his wife is experiencing. In our culture, a father-to-be may experience nausea, headache, back and muscle aches, insomnia, fatigue and depression.

I recently read that reproduction and fetal development may be affected if a man is exposed to various chemicals. Is this true?
Yes. Exposure by the father-to-be to alcohol, cigarettes, certain drugs and some environmental hazards could harm the unborn baby. This could also affect the man's ability to father a child.

What kind of problems can be caused by a man's exposure to these substances?
Problems include miscarriage, stillbirth, birth defects, low birth weight babies, a greater risk of childhood cancer and even subtle learning disabilities.

When is this exposure the most important?
Usually male exposure is harmful if it occurs before and around the time of conception. However, we also know that a father-to-be's smoking during pregnancy has been linked to various problems.

I've heard that my husband's use of alcohol before my pregnancy may have an effect on the baby. In what way?
Some researchers believe heavy alcohol consumption by the baby's father may produce *fetal alcohol syndrome* (FAS) in the baby. See Chapter 13 for further information on FAS. Alcohol intake by the father has also been linked to intra-uterine growth retardation.

My partner has used 'recreational drugs' from time to time. I think he was using them when I got pregnant. Is this going to cause any problems?
Your partner's drug habits may have an effect on your pregnancy. The best thing to do is to tell your doctor and see if there is anything that can be done to reassure you about the well-being of your baby.

Is it true I need to be concerned about substances my partner is exposed to at work?
Yes. Substances may be brought into your home on your partner's work clothes. If you think you may be exposed to hazardous substances in this manner, be sure to discuss it with your partner and your doctor.

I don't smoke, but my partner does. Should I try to get him to stop now that I'm pregnant?
When a non-smoking pregnant woman and her unborn baby are exposed to secondary smoke, both are exposed to chemicals that can harm them. It is a good idea to ask your partner to stop smoking during your pregnancy or at least not to smoke inside your home.

My partner is 53. Can his age cause problems for me or my baby?
We now have information indicating the age and health of the father of your baby *does* make a difference to the health of your baby. Some researchers believe there may be an increased risk of Down's syndrome if the baby's father is over 50.

My husband and I have talked about having him cut the umbilical cord after the baby is born. Will the doctor let him do this?
Cutting the cord is something many men enjoy doing. Talk to your doctor about your husband's participation in the delivery.

I'm afraid I'm going to feel exhausted dealing with the baby after we get home. How can I get my husband to help me?
It's better when both partners share the responsibilities and chores of parenthood. Form an equal-parenthood partnership with your husband, and encourage him to take equal responsibility for parenting your new baby. He'll enjoy being a father much more if he is actively involved in the care and decision-making for his new daughter or son.

My doctor said my husband can be very important to me during labour and delivery. How?

Your husband can help in many ways. He can help prepare you for labour and delivery and can support you as you labour. He can share in the joy of the delivery of your baby. He can also support you emotionally, which can be very important to you both.

CHAPTER 12

Sexually Transmitted Diseases

I've heard sexually transmitted diseases can harm a growing baby. Is this true?
A *sexually transmitted disease (STD)* can harm a developing fetus. If you have an STD, you must be treated as soon as possible!

What exactly is a sexually transmitted disease?
A sexually transmitted disease is a disease that is contracted during sexual activity, whether it is sexual intercourse, oral intercourse or anal intercourse.

What are some of the STDs that I need to be aware of?
The most common sexually transmitted diseases include:

. candidal vulvovaginitis
. trichomonal vaginitis
. condyloma acuminatum (venereal warts)
. genital herpes simplex infection
. chlamydia
. gonorrhoea
. syphilis
. Aids

What is candidal vulvovaginitis?
Candidal vulvovaginitis is an infection caused by yeast, or monilia, and usually affects the vagina and vulva. Yeast infections are more common in pregnant women than in non-pregnant women.

What kind of problems can yeast infections cause during pregnancy?
This STD has no major negative effects on pregnancy, but it can cause discomfort and anxiety for you.

How are yeast infections treated during pregnancy?
Yeast infections are harder to control when you are pregnant. They may require frequent retreatment or longer treatment (10–14 days instead of 3–7 days). Creams or suppositories used for treatment are safe during pregnancy. Your partner does not have to be treated unless he has symptoms.

I've heard of a new medication that I only have to take once, orally, to clear up a yeast infection. Can it be taken during pregnancy?
You're talking about fluconazole (Diflucan) a new anti-fungal drug. You take it orally, just once, to treat a yeast infection. We are not recommending it during pregnancy or lactation because it has not yet been proved safe for use in either situation.

What kind of problems can a yeast infection cause the baby?
A newborn baby can get *thrush* (a mouth infection) after passing through a birth canal infected with a yeast infection. Treatment of the newborn baby with nystatin is effective.

What is trichomonal vaginitis?
Trichomonal vaginitis is an infection caused by parasites called *trichomonas*. Symptoms include persistent burning and itching of the vulva area accompanied by a frothy white or yellow discharge.

What kind of problems can trichomonal vaginitis cause during pregnancy?
There is some evidence that it predisposes to premature labour.

Is treatment of trichomonal vaginitis a concern during pregnancy?
Some doctors thought metronidazole, the drug usually used to treat trichomonal vaginitis, might be harmful to the fetus. However, there was never any evidence for this, but as a matter of general principle, treatment may be deferred until the second trimester if the infection is not causing significant symptoms.

What are condylomata acuminatum (venereal warts)?
Condylomata acuminatum are skin tags or warts that are transmitted by sexual contact.

What causes condylomata?
Condylomata are caused by a virus called the *human papillomavirus (HPV)*, which is passed during intercourse.

Why are venereal warts a problem during pregnancy?
Warty skin tags often become enlarged during pregnancy and have been known to block the vagina at the time of delivery. If a woman has extensive venereal warts, a caesarean section may be necessary to avoid heavy bleeding and other complications.

How can venereal warts affect a baby?
Infants delivered through a birth canal infected with venereal warts have been known to get laryngeal papillomas (small benign tumours on the vocal cords) after delivery.

Can venereal warts be treated during pregnancy?
Often they can be. Doctors use several methods to treat them, including freezing the warts off, laser treatment and chemical removal. If warts become large enough to interfere with delivery, your physician may recommend removing them. With the exception of one chemical

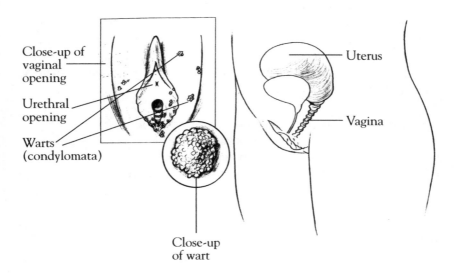

Close-up of vaginal opening

Urethral opening

Warts (condylomata)

Close-up of wart

Uterus

Vagina

Condylomata (venereal warts) can cause problems during pregnancy.

irritant, podophyllin, all three treatment methods have been safely used during pregnancy.

What is genital herpes simplex infection?
Genital herpes simplex infection is a herpes simplex infection involving the genital area. It can be significant during pregnancy because of the danger of infecting a newborn baby with the disease at the time of delivery.

What are the symptoms of genital herpes?
Usually clusters of small blisters appear in the genital area within a week after infection. At first the blisters are itchy, then they become painful and break, leaving painful ulcers. Symptoms can also include aches and pains, fatigue, fever and a vaginal discharge. These symptoms usually disappear within three weeks. Subsequent outbreaks can occur at any time, but are usually shorter and milder.

What kind of problems can herpes cause a mother-to-be?
Infection early in pregnancy may be associated with an increase in miscarriage or premature delivery.

What kind of problems can herpes cause the baby?
Infection in the mother is associated with low birth weight in the baby. We believe an infant can contract the infection from travelling through an infected birth canal. When membranes rupture, the infection may also travel upward to the uterus and infect the baby. This could result in fetal infections. Infected newborn babies have a mortality rate of 50 per cent.

How can herpes simplex be treated during pregnancy?
There is no effective treatment. Acyclovir may decrease the symptoms, but the safety of acyclovir in pregnancy has not been established beyond all doubt. When a woman has an active herpes infection late in pregnancy, a caesarean section may be performed to prevent the baby from travelling through the infected birth canal.

If I have herpes, can I prevent my baby from becoming infected?
If you have an outbreak at the time of delivery, a caesarean section is often done to protect the baby from exposure.

How can I avoid getting genital herpes?

You must know your partner is free from infection. If your partner suspects he has herpes, he should see a doctor for treatment. If your partner has herpes or could have been exposed to it, the best way to avoid the disease is through abstinence from sex during outbreaks and having him wear a condom during intercourse.

What is chlamydia?

Chlamydia is a common sexually transmitted disease. It is estimated that between 3 and 5 million people are infected each year. Symptoms include vaginal discharge and pelvic pain. However, it can be symptomless – you may not know you have been exposed. Between 20 and 40 per cent of all sexually active women have been exposed at some time.

How can chlamydia affect pregnancy?

One of the most important complications of chlamydia is *pelvic inflammatory disease (PID)*, which is a severe infection of the female organs. If you have had PID, your chance of having an ectopic pregnancy is greater. During pregnancy, a mother-to-be can pass a chlamydial infection to her baby as it travels through the birth canal. The baby will have a 20–50 per cent chance of getting chlamydia.

How does a chlamydial infection affect the baby?

A baby exposed to chlamydia may be born with an eye infection or pneumonia.

If chlamydia is often symptomless, how will I know I have it?

Tests that can be done for chlamydia include a pelvic examination and a swab from the canal of the cervix.

How is chlamydia treated?

Treatment of chlamydia usually involves tetracycline, which should not be given to a pregnant woman. During pregnancy, erythromycin is the drug of choice.

What is gonorrhoea?

Gonorrhoea is a venereal infection transmitted primarily by sexual intercourse. In a woman, the urethra, vulva, vagina and fallopian tubes may be involved. There may be no symptoms of the disease.

How can gonorrhoea affect the baby?

The baby may be infected as it passes through the birth canal, resulting in severe conjunctivitis (eye inflammation). Eyedrops are given to newborn babies to prevent this problem. Other infections in the baby may also occur.

How is gonorrhoea treated during pregnancy?

Gonorrhoeal infections are easily treated with penicillin and other antibiotics that are safe to use during pregnancy.

What is syphilis?

Syphilis is a sexually transmitted disease characterised by lesions that may involve any organ or tissue. The disease may be present for years without symptoms.

How can syphilis affect a pregnancy?

Syphilis increases the chance of stillbirth. It can also cause infection in the newborn's lungs, liver, spleen, pancreas or other organs. Any stage of syphilis during pregnancy can result in infection in an infant.

How can syphilis be treated during pregnancy?

Syphilis can be treated effectively during pregnancy with penicillin and other drugs that are safe to use.

I know that Aids affects more women today. In addition to the personal issue, why is this important to a pregnant woman?

Pregnancy may hide some of the symptoms of Aids (acquired immune deficiency syndrome), which can make the disease harder to discover. Some possible treatments may not be used during pregnancy.

Can a woman infected with Aids pass it to her baby?

It is possible for a woman to pass HIV, the virus that causes Aids, to the baby before birth, during birth and, if she breast feeds, after birth. The survival rate for children diagnosed with Aids in the first 6 months of life is low.

How can a woman find out if she has Aids or is positive for HIV?

Two blood tests are used – the ELISA test and the Western Blot test. If the ELISA test is positive, it is confirmed by the Western Blot test. Both tests measure antibodies to the virus, not the virus itself. No test should be considered positive unless the Western Blot test is done – it is believed to be 99 per cent sensitive and specific.

I just heard about a new treatment plan for pregnant women who have Aids. If a woman is given AZT during her pregnancy, the baby almost always will be born without Aids. Is this true?
The risk to a baby infected with the HIV virus is serious and significant, but advances continue to be made in Aids research. Recent research has shown that AZT treatment can decrease the likelihood that an infected mother will pass the infection to her baby. If you are concerned about HIV and Aids, discuss it with your doctor.

CHAPTER 13

Substance Use and Abuse

Can the substances I take affect my developing baby?
Yes, they can and do. It's *never* too early to start thinking about how your actions affect the baby growing inside you. Some substances that you can use safely may have adverse effects on a developing fetus. Other substances are bad for both you and your baby.

What kind of activities can affect my baby?
Just about anything you do can affect your baby. Cigarette smoke, alcohol, drugs, tranquillisers, even caffeine can affect a fetus. (For a discussion of caffeine, see Chapter 5.)

How do researchers know that these substances affect a developing baby?
Information about the effects of specific substances on a human pregnancy often comes from cases of exposure before the pregnancy is discovered. These cases help researchers understand possible harmful effects, but they don't help us to understand the picture completely. For this reason, we cannot make exact statements about particular substances and their effects on the mother or developing baby.

Cigarette Smoking

I smoke cigarettes every day. Should I stop?
Yes! A pregnant woman who smokes one pack of cigarettes a day (20 cigarettes) inhales tobacco smoke more than 11,000 times during an average pregnancy! Tobacco smoke inhaled by the mother *can* affect a growing baby.

Why is cigarette smoking so harmful?
Tobacco smoke inhaled by the mother contains many harmful substances, including nicotine, carbon monoxide, hydrogen cyanide, tars, resins and some cancer-causing agents. When a pregnant woman inhales cigarette smoke, these chemicals pass through the placenta to the developing baby.

What kind of effects will my cigarette smoking have on the baby?
Infants born to mothers who smoke weigh less than other babies. This can cause problems for the baby. Lower IQ scores and increased incidence of reading disorders have been noted in children born to mothers who smoked during pregnancy. Hyperactivity is also more common in babies born to women who smoked. Research has shown that smoking during pregnancy interferes with the body's absorption of vitamins B and C and folic acid, and increases the risk of pregnancy-related complications.

I've heard pregnancy complications can increase for the mother-to-be if she smokes. Is that true?
Yes. Smoking increases the incidence of serious complications for the pregnant woman. The risk of developing placental abruption increases almost 25 per cent in moderate smokers and 65 per cent in heavy smokers. Placenta praevia occurs 25 per cent more often in moderate smokers and 90 per cent more often in heavy smokers. For further information on these problems, see Chapter 15.

In addition, cigarette smoking during pregnancy increases the risk of miscarriage, death of the fetus or death of a baby soon after birth. This risk is directly related to the number of cigarettes a woman smokes each day. It can increase as much as 35 per cent for a woman who smokes more than a packet of cigarettes a day.

What can I do about it if I smoke?
The best way you can help yourself is to quit smoking completely before and during your pregnancy. If you can't do this – it's hard to stop suddenly – reduce the number of cigarettes you smoke. It may help reduce your risks.

I don't smoke, but my husband does. Will this hurt me or the baby?
Some research suggests a non-smoker and her unborn baby who are exposed to secondary smoke are exposed to carboxyhaemoglobin and nicotine. These substances may harm you or your baby. It is a good idea

to ask your husband to stop smoking while you are pregnant. You might suggest he stops smoking altogether.

Alcohol Use

Is it all right to drink alcohol while I'm pregnant?

Alcohol use by a pregnant woman carries some risk. Even moderate use of alcohol has been linked to an increase in the chance of miscarriage. Excessive alcohol consumption during pregnancy can result in abnormalities in the baby. Chronic heavy use of alcohol during pregnancy can lead to *fetal alcohol syndrome*, which is abnormal fetal development.

What is fetal alcohol syndrome?

Fetal alcohol syndrome (FAS) is a collection of problems that affect children born to alcoholic women. It is characterised by growth retardation before and after birth. Defects in the heart and limbs and unusual facial characteristics, such as a short, upturned nose, a flat upper jawbone and 'different' eyes, have also been seen in FAS children. These children may also have behavioural problems, impaired speech and impaired use of joints and muscles.

How much alcohol is 'too much'?

At this time, some doctors believe *any* amount of alcohol is too much. Most studies indicate four to five drinks a day are required to cause FAS, but mild abnormalities have been said to be associated with as little as two drinks a day (1oz of alcohol). It's best to avoid alcohol completely while you're pregnant.

I don't drink much. Can I drink socially while I'm pregnant?

There is a lot of disagreement about this because we do not know what is a 'safe' level of alcohol consumption during pregnancy. I recommend not drinking any alcohol during pregnancy. Why take the risk of harming your baby?

What about drinking before pregnancy, while I'm trying to get pregnant?

If you're trying to get pregnant, you probably won't know exactly when you do conceive. Why take chances? It's a good idea to stop drinking while you are trying to conceive – that way you'll avoid any alcohol-related problems.

I've heard that drugs taken with alcohol can cause more problems. How is that?
If drugs are taken with alcohol, it increases the chance of damaging the fetus. Drugs that cause the greatest concern include pain-relieving drugs, anti-depressants and anti-convulsants.

I read somewhere that my partner's use of alcohol before my pregnancy may affect the fetus. Is this true?
Some researchers believe heavy alcohol consumption by the baby's father may produce fetal alcohol syndrome in the baby. Alcohol intake by the father has also been linked to intra-uterine growth retardation.

Should I take any other precautions with regards to alcohol?
Be very careful about substances you use that may contain alcohol. Over-the-counter cough medicines and cold remedies often contain alcohol – as much as 25 per cent!

Drug Use and Drug Abuse

I want to know more about drug use, drug abuse and pregnancy. First, how do you define 'drug abuse'?
Drug abuse usually refers to drugs prohibited by law, but it can also include use of legal substances, such as alcohol, caffeine and tobacco. Legal medicines, such as benzodiazepine or barbiturates, may also have harmful effects, whether they are used for legitimate or illegal reasons.

What is 'physical dependence'?
Physical dependence implies the drug must be taken to avoid unpleasant withdrawal symptoms – it does not always mean addiction or drug abuse. For example, many caffeine users develop withdrawal symptoms if they stop drinking coffee, but they are not considered drug abusers or drug addicts.

What is 'psychological dependence'?
Psychological dependence means the user has developed an emotional need for a drug or medicine. This need may be more compelling than a physical need and can provide the stimulus for continued drug use.

Can the use of drugs impact on my pregnancy?

Yes! Certain drugs damage the developing fetus. In addition, a woman who abuses drugs often has more complications in pregnancy because of her lifestyle.

What kind of problems do you mean?

With the use of certain substances, nutritional deficiencies are common. Anaemia and fetal growth retardation can also occur. A pregnant woman may have an increased chance of toxaemia or pre-eclampsia.

What about marijuana use during pregnancy? Can it hurt the baby?

Marijuana (hashish) contains tetrahydrocannabinol (THC). Research has shown that the use of marijuana by a mother-to-be can cause problems including attention deficits, memory problems and impaired decision making in children; these appear between the ages 3 and 12.

How do amphetamines affect the baby?

Some researchers have thought that the use during pregnancy of central nervous system stimulants, such as amphetamines, is associated with an increase in cardiovascular defects in babies.

Some women use barbiturates. Are these harmful during pregnancy?

Barbiturate use may be associated with birth defects, although this has not been proved definitely. However, we have seen withdrawal, poor feeding, seizures and other problems in babies born to mothers who abused barbiturates during pregnancy.

Can other tranquillisers affect a pregnant woman?

Tranquillising agents include benzodiazepines (Valium and Librium) and other, newer agents. Several studies have related the use of these drugs to an increase in congenital malformations, but others have found no harm in them.

What are opioids?

Opioids are derived from opium and synthetic compounds with similar actions. They produce euphoria, drowsiness or sleepiness, and decreased sensitivity to pain. Habitual use can lead to physical dependence.

What common drugs are opioids?
Opioids include morphine, pethidine, heroin and codeine.

What kind of problems can opioids cause?
These drugs are associated with a variety of congenital abnormalities and complications in pregnancy. Women who use opioids during pregnancy are often at high risk of premature labour, intra-uterine growth retardation and pre-eclampsia.

What can happen to a baby if the mother uses opioids?
A baby born to a mother who uses opioids may experience withdrawal symptoms after birth.

Are there any other problems associated with using opioids during pregnancy?
If the mother uses the drugs intravenously, other problems may occur, such as Aids, hepatitis and endocarditis. Any of these is considered *very* serious during pregnancy.

Is the use of hallucinogens declining?
The use of some hallucinogens, such as LSD, mescaline and peyote, is not as common as it was several years ago. However, phencyclidine (PCP) is a powerful hallucinogen whose use is growing.

How does the use of PCP affect a pregnancy?
PCP, also called *angel dust*, can cause severe mental illness and loss of contact with reality in the mother. Research has shown it causes abnormal development in some humans, so we believe it can cause abnormal development in human babies, although it has not been definitely proved.

I know cocaine use is more common today. How does it affect a pregnancy?
Today, use of cocaine is a more common complication of pregnancy. Often a user consumes the drug over a long period of time, such as several days. During this time, the user may eat or drink very little, which can have serious consequences for a developing fetus.

How does cocaine affect the mother-to-be?
Use of cocaine has been associated with convulsions, arrhythmias, hypertension and hyperthermia in a pregnant woman. Continual use

of cocaine can affect maternal nutrition and temperature control, which can harm the fetus. Cocaine use has been linked with miscarriage, placental abruption and congenital defects.

I've heard that the use of cocaine during early pregnancy can cause serious problems. Is this true?

If a woman uses cocaine during the first 12 weeks of pregnancy, there is an increased risk of miscarriage. Damage to the developing baby can occur as early as 3 *days* after conception!

How does cocaine use by the mother-to-be affect the baby?

Infants born to mothers who use cocaine during pregnancy often have lower intelligence and long term mental deficiencies. Sudden infant death syndrome (SIDS) is also more common in these babies. Some babies are stillborn.

What about crack use?

All that I have stated about cocaine use can be applied to the use of crack.

I know someone who used drugs a few times while she was pregnant. Her baby seems all right. Aren't you exaggerating the dangers?

No. Your friend was lucky. A fetus is totally dependent on the mother-to-be for all its needs, so everything a mother-to-be does can affect her baby. What may seem like a small amount to a woman can have a major effect on the fetus whose organs are still being formed. It is up to you to do all you can to help your baby have the best possible start in life.

CHAPTER 14

Special Concerns of the Single Mother-to-be

I've included this chapter in the book because many women today are having their babies alone, either by choice or because the baby's father is unwilling or unable to be with them. Others will have the support of the father-to-be, but have decided not to get married. My goal in writing it is to give you a foundation for seeking information about your unique situation. I feel comfortable answering the first group of questions because I have been asked many of them before.

I have not answered the second group of questions because they concern legal matters that I am not qualified to answer. However, they are included because there are many legal ramifications involved. I hope you will use the questions to help formulate questions about your personal situation to ask your solicitor, a hospital social worker, your doctor or family members.

I'm a single woman who has chosen to have her baby alone. What should I tell people who ask me why I am doing this?
It doesn't matter what people ask you – really it's none of their business. What is important is how you feel about the pregnancy. It's up to you to decide what you want to tell people and how much of an explanation you want to provide.

Some people think I'm mad to have a baby alone. What should I say to them?
Your friends won't treat you this way. Once they understand your situation, they will support you. If others give you a hard time, don't talk to them about your pregnancy or your reasons for having your baby alone.

I feel as if I have no one close to share my pregnancy problems and concerns with. What can I do?

Share your problems and concerns with your family and friends. Mothers of young children can identify with your experiences – they had the same or similar experiences recently. If you have friends or family members who have young children, talk to them. Even if you were married and living with your husband, you would probably share your concerns with all of these people. Try not to let your situation alter this.

My family is against my decision to have my baby alone. Is there anything I can do about this?

If this is a decision you are comfortable with, deal with their discomfort by asking them to talk about the reasons they are against your pregnancy. You will never change some people's minds, so you will have to learn to live with their disapproval or ignore it.

Some people seem very interested in my situation but hesitate to talk to me. Should I encourage them to ask questions?

Only if you are comfortable with their questions. Some people are genuinely concerned about you; others are just nosy. Before you answer, decide if the people are truly interested in you. Then share with them as much or as little as you are comfortable discussing.

I've having a lot of trouble emotionally with this pregnancy. Who should I talk to about it?

Begin by talking to your doctor. He or she can direct you to a counsellor or a support group, depending on what you need.

Will I have to make special plans for when I go into labour? What should they cover?

Just as any pregnant woman does, you must decide who will be with you when you labour and deliver, and who will be there to help afterwards. The only special plan I can think of is to decide how you will get to the hospital. One woman decided to have her friend drive her, but couldn't reach her in time. Her next option (all part of her plan) was to call a taxi, which got her to the hospital in plenty of time.

I don't have a particular person in mind to ask – what can I do about someone to be with me in labour?
Ask a good friend, a relative or someone else who is close to you. Not all women have their partner with them. I've often found that a woman who has already given birth under similar conditions is an excellent companion. She will understand your discomfort and be able to identify with your experience.

If I am a single mother, will the midwives treat me differently?
In all my experiences in medical school, during my residency and in my practice, the nurses and midwives I have dealt with have been professionals. Their job is to provide the best care they possibly can, and they pride themselves in taking care of their patients. I have never known any of them to treat anyone differently for any reason.

How will it be different for me when I take my baby home by myself?
A new baby is always an incredible challenge, in any situation. You will probably need more support from family and friends because you will not have anyone to share the responsibilities with at home. Don't hesitate to ask for their assistance. If you have no one you can ask to give of their time, you might consider hiring someone to stay with you at night for the first week or two, to allow you to get back on your feet.

Do you think people will treat me or my baby differently because I am a single mother?
Today, being a single mother isn't that unusual. Many women of all ages have made this decision. Some people may treat you differently; others won't care. Good friends and family members should draw closer to you.

Because I had donor insemination, my baby won't have another set of grandparents, aunts and uncles. Do you think this will be a problem?
Families today are different from the way they were in the past. Many children don't have a complete set of parents or grandparents, even in the closest family units. I've found in these situations that an older family friend can be just as loving and giving to a child as a grandparent. Encourage older friends to take an active part in your child's life.

Are there support groups for single parents?
Yes, there are. Ask your doctor or midwife for the names of groups in your area.

I'm scared that if I get sick, no one will be there to take care of my baby. How can I deal with this problem?
You need to plan ahead for this situation. Find a family member or close friend who can be called upon to help out in case this happens. Knowing you have provided for this event should give you peace of mind.

People seem to assume my partner and I are married, but we aren't. What should we do about this?
If you are pregnant and you are together, most people will assume you are married. First, decide if it's important to clear up the misunderstanding. If it's a sales clerk or a waitress who makes this assumption, then it probably isn't important to say anything. If it's your doctor, you should let him or her know what is going on.

Other Questions

The following questions are included without answers because they are legal questions that should be discussed with a solicitor who specialises in family law. Use them as a guide to developing the questions you need to ask about your particular situation.

I've heard that if I'm unmarried I have to get a special birth certificate. Is that true?

I'm having my baby alone, and I'm concerned about who can make medical decisions for me and the baby. Is there anything I can do about this concern?

I'm not married, but I am deeply involved with my baby's father. Can my partner make medical decisions for me if I have problems during or after the birth?

If anything happens to me, can my partner make medical decisions for our baby after it is born?

What are the legal rights of my baby's father if we are not married?

Do my partner's parents also have legal rights in regard to my child (their grandchild)?

My baby's father and I went our separate ways before I knew I was pregnant. Do I have to tell him about the baby?

I chose to have donor (artificial) insemination. If anything happens to me during my labour or delivery, who can make medical decisions for me?

Who can make medical decisions for my baby?

I got pregnant by donor insemination. What do I put on the birth certificate under 'father's name'?

Is there any way I can find out more about my sperm donor's family medical history?

Will the sperm bank send me updates if medical problems appear in my sperm donor's family?

I had donor insemination. Does the baby's father have any legal right to be part of my child's life in the future?

Someone was joking with me that my child could marry its sister or brother some day (because I had donor insemination) and wouldn't even know it. Is this possible?

As my child grows up, he or she may need some sort of medical help (like a donor kidney) from a sibling. Will the sperm bank give out this kind of information?

CHAPTER 15

Problems and Warning Signs

I'm worried that I won't know when to call my doctor if there are problems during my pregnancy. Are there warning signs I should know about?

If you think there is something to worry about, don't be afraid to ask for help. General warning signs include the following:

- vaginal bleeding
- painful urination
- severe abdominal pain
- loss of fluid from the vagina, usually a gushing of fluid, but sometimes a trickle or continual wetness
- a big change in the movement of the baby or a lack of fetal movement
- high fever (more than 100.6°F/38.0°C)
- chills
- severe vomiting or inability to keep food or liquids down
- blurring of vision
- severe swelling of the face or fingers
- a severe headache or a headache that won't go away
- an injury or accident serious enough to give you concern about the well-being of your pregnancy, such as a fall or a car accident

Bleeding during Pregnancy

I'm 7 weeks pregnant and started to bleed a little last night. It scares me. What should I do?
Tell your doctor about any bleeding; he or she may want you to have an ultrasound scan. This early in pregnancy you are probably worrying about having a miscarriage. Be assured that bleeding during pregnancy is not unusual and doesn't always mean a problem. About one woman in five bleeds sometime in early pregnancy.

What causes the bleeding?
Usually we cannot give a definite answer as to what causes it, but we do know that it is *not* usually a problem. If you experience any vaginal bleeding during pregnancy, call your doctor.

I rang my doctor and told her I had some bleeding, and she told me to rest and not to have intercourse. Isn't there some medicine I can take or something I can do to stop the bleeding and make sure everything is going to be all right?
You doctor gave you good advice – there isn't any surgery or medicine that will stop the bleeding. If your concern or your doctor's concern is high, she may schedule you for an ultrasound scan. A scan won't stop anything from happening; it may give some reassurance, but you may still bleed. Decisions about a course of treatment or actions to take are very individual and must be discussed with your doctor, who knows your past history and individual situation.

If I am bleeding and go to bed to try to rest, will that help?
If you have any bleeding, contact your doctor before you do anything. Follow his or her instructions. Going to bed and resting may help. Your doctor knows your medical and pregnancy history, so follow his or her advice.

Falling while you're Pregnant

What should I do if I fall?
If you fall, contact your doctor; you may require attention. If it's a bad fall, your doctor may advise monitoring the baby's heartbeat or having an ultrasound scan.

I fell down today. How can I be sure that my baby wasn't hurt?
A fall is the most frequent cause of minor injury during pregnancy. Fortunately, a fall is usually without serious injury to the fetus or to the mother. Even if it was only a minor fall, however, you should still get in touch with your doctor.

If I fall, are there problems or warning signs I should look for?
Some signs and symptoms to alert you to a possible problem include:

- bleeding
- a gush of fluid from the vagina, indicating rupture of membranes
- severe abdominal pain

Movement of the baby after a fall is reassuring.

Miscarriages

This is my first pregnancy, and I'm very nervous about having a miscarriage. What exactly is a miscarriage?
A *miscarriage* means losing the pregnancy before 20 weeks. An embryo or a fetus is delivered before it can survive outside the womb. This may also be called a *spontaneous abortion*.

Why do miscarriages occur?
Most of the time we don't know – a miscarriage can happen for many different reasons. The most common finding in early miscarriages is an abnormality in the development of the early embryo. Research indicates that more than half of these miscarriages have chromosomal abnormalities. Outside factors, called *teratogens*, can cause miscarriage, and maternal factors are also believed to be relevant in some miscarriages.

Do miscarriages occur very often?
It has been estimated that as many 50 per cent of pregnancies miscarry after implantation in the uterus, but most of these are unrecognised and ascribed to a 'heavy period'. Of pregnancies recognised after about 6 weeks from the last menstrual period, only 7 to 10 per cent miscarry.

What kind of 'outside factors' can cause a miscarriage?
Research has shown that radiation and some chemicals (drugs or medications) may cause a miscarriage.

What 'maternal factors' can cause a miscarriage?
There are many maternal factors that can result in a miscarriage.

- Research has shown that unusual infections in the mother-to-be, such as listeria, toxoplasmosis and syphilis, may cause miscarriage.
- A deficiency of progesterone is believed by some doctors to be a cause of early miscarriage.
- Genital infections have been shown to trigger miscarriage. When an infection is found, the woman and her partner are treated.
- Sometimes a woman's body makes antibodies that attack the fetus or disrupt the function of the placenta.
- Women who smoke have a higher rate of miscarriage.
- Alcohol has also been blamed for an increased rate of miscarriage.

I've heard that sometimes a particular couple can have a high risk of a miscarriage. Can you explain this?
This does cause some confusion for many people, but it is fairly easy to understand. When their genes unite upon fertilisation of the egg by the sperm, the union may produce genetic abnormalities that can cause a miscarriage. Genetic screening can sometimes reveal this. In other cases, observation of fertilisation in the test tube – *in vitro* fertilisation – may show a defect.

Can nutrient deficiency cause a miscarriage?
We have no concrete evidence that deficiency of any particular nutrient or even moderate deficiency of all nutrients can cause a miscarriage.

Can a woman cause a miscarriage to occur?
Not usually, so don't blame yourself if you have a miscarriage. It's a normal reaction to look for a reason for losing a pregnancy and to think you might have done something wrong. Many women try to blame stress, emotional upset or physical activity for causing a miscarriage. These things do not usually cause miscarriages.

I've heard that there are different types of miscarriage. What does this mean?
The medical descriptions for different types of miscarriage include:

- threatened miscarriage
- inevitable miscarriage
- incomplete miscarriage

- missed abortion
- habitual abortion

What is a 'threatened miscarriage'?

A *threatened miscarriage* occurs when there is a bloody discharge from the vagina during the first half of pregnancy. Bleeding may last for days or weeks. There may or may not be cramping and pain that may feel like a menstrual cramp or mild backache. Bed rest is about all a woman can do to try to prevent the miscarriage from happening, although being active does not itself cause miscarriage.

What is an 'inevitable miscarriage'?

An *inevitable miscarriage* occurs with the rupture of membranes, dilatation of the cervix and passage of blood clots and even tissue. Loss of the pregnancy is almost certain under these circumstances. Contraction of the uterus usually occurs, expelling the embryo or products of conception.

What is an 'incomplete miscarriage'?

In an *incomplete miscarriage*, the entire pregnancy is not immediately expelled. Part of the pregnancy may be passed while the rest remains in the uterus. Bleeding may be heavy and continues until the uterus is empty or is emptied by a doctor with the patient under an anaesthetic.

What is a 'missed miscarriage'?

A *missed miscarriage* can occur when an embryo that has died earlier is retained in the uterus. A woman may not bleed or have any other symptoms. The period between the failure of the pregnancy and the discovery of the miscarriage may be weeks.

What is 'habitual miscarriage'?

Habitual miscarriage usually refers to three or more consecutive miscarriages.

What are the warning signs of a miscarriage?

The first warning sign is bleeding from the vagina, followed by cramping. Call your doctor if you experience these problems! The longer you bleed and cramp, the more likely you are to have a miscarriage.

What can I do if I think I'm having a miscarriage?
Talk to your doctor. In nearly all instances, there is nothing you can do to stop a miscarriage from happening. There is no surgery that can be done or medicine you can take to stop a miscarriage. Most physicians recommend bed rest and decreased activity. Some recommend use of a hormone called *progesterone*, but not all agree that it is of any value. Ultrasound scans and blood tests may be used to assist your doctor in determining whether you are going to miscarry, but you may have to wait and see.

What will my doctor do if I am having a miscarriage?
If you expel all of the products of the pregnancy and bleeding stops and cramping goes away, you may be done with it. If everything is not expelled, it will be necessary to perform a D and C (dilatation and curettage), which is minor surgery to empty the uterus. It is preferable to do this surgery so you won't bleed for a long time, risking anaemia and infection.

I've heard a woman needs to be concerned about rhesus sensitisation if she has a miscarriage. Is this true?
If you're rhesus negative and have a miscarriage, you will need to receive anti-D immunoglobulin. This applies *only* if you are rhesus negative.

If I have a miscarriage, will there be an embryo or a fetus? What will it look like?
You usually won't see a fetus. What you pass appears to be white, grey or red tissue and will look like a piece of placenta.

If I miscarry, will it be possible to tell if it was a boy or girl?
No, this is not possible.

When my sister had a miscarriage, they told her to save the tissue, but she had already flushed it. Why did they want her to save it?
Some doctors want you to bring the tissue to the lab to verify it was really the pregnancy that was passed and not just a blood clot.

My friend had a miscarriage when she was 3 months pregnant, and she blames herself. Is this possible?
A woman shouldn't blame herself or her partner for a miscarriage. It is usually impossible to look back at everything a woman did, ate or was

exposed to and find the cause of a miscarriage. Remember, usually no reason can be found for a miscarriage.

If I am having a miscarriage, will my pregnancy test be positive?
Yes. The hormones will make your pregnancy test positive.

A friend of mine had a stillbirth last year. What's the difference between a miscarriage and a stillbirth?
In medical terms, loss of the fetus before 20 weeks is a *miscarriage*. Loss of the fetus after 20 weeks is a *stillbirth*.

Ectopic Pregnancy

What is an ectopic pregnancy?
Ectopic pregnancy, sometimes called a *tubal pregnancy*, is not common. It occurs about once in every 100 pregnancies. An ectopic pregnancy happens when implantation occurs *outside* the uterine cavity, usually in the fallopian tube.

I'm 8 weeks pregnant and have pain on my side where I think my ovary is. Could it be an ectopic pregnancy?
It isn't unusual to have mild pain early in pregnancy from a cyst on the ovary or stretching of the uterus or ligaments. It probably isn't an ectopic pregnancy, but if the pain is bad enough to cause you concern, call your doctor.

What are the factors that increase the risk of having an ectopic pregnancy?
There are quite a few factors that can increase the risk of an ectopic pregnancy, including:

• pelvic infections (PID or pelvic inflammatory disease)
• previous ruptured appendix
• previous ectopic pregnancy
• surgery on your fallopian tubes (such as reversal of a tubal ligation)
• use of an intra-uterine contraceptive device

How is an ectopic pregnancy diagnosed?
Diagnosis of an ectopic pregnancy can be difficult and may require a couple of tests and some waiting. Tests include ultrasound scanning,

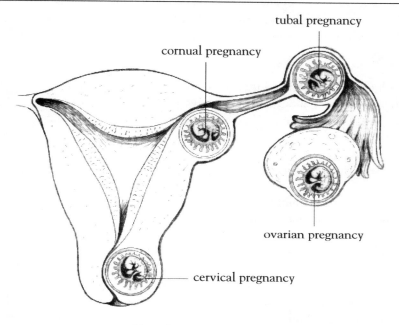

Sites of ectopic pregnancies.

quantitative HCGs and laparoscopy (a visual examination inside the abdomen). Even with these tests, it may be a few days or weeks before a definitive diagnosis can be made.

I've had some pain and bleeding, and my doctor is concerned about an ectopic pregnancy. Yesterday I had a quantitative HCG, and I'm supposed to have another one tomorrow. What is a quantitative HCG?

A *quantitative* HCG (*human chorionic gonadotrophin*) is a special pregnancy test done on your blood. HCG is a hormone produced during pregnancy; it increases very rapidly early in pregnancy. A regular pregnancy test, using blood or urine, gives you a positive or negative ('yes' or 'no') answer. A quantitative HCG assigns a number to indicate how pregnant you are. The numbers aren't exact, but in a normal pregnancy they increase in a way that can help your doctor decide if it is a normal pregnancy. This test is not used in normal pregnancies but can be very helpful when you are concerned about a miscarriage or ectopic pregnancy.

If I have an ectopic pregnancy, will a pregnancy test be positive?
Yes. The hormones produced with an ectopic pregnancy still make your pregnancy test positive.

If I have an ectopic pregnancy, what can the doctors do for me?
An ectopic pregnancy almost always requires surgery to correct the problem, which results in loss of the pregnancy.

Blood Clots during Pregnancy

My sister has thrombophlebitis during her pregnancy. Is that the same as a blood clot in the leg?
Yes, it is. The problem has several names, including *venous thrombosis, thromboembolic disease, thrombophlebitis* and *deep vein thrombosis*.

Why do blood clots in the leg occur in pregnancy?
This condition is more likely to occur during pregnancy because of the changes in blood circulation. There is a slowing of blood flow in the legs because of pressure from the uterus on blood vessels and because of changes in the blood and its clotting mechanisms. Blood clots occur in less than 1 per cent of all pregnancies.

What causes blood clots during pregnancy?
The most likely cause of a blood clot in the legs during pregnancy is decreased blood flow, called *stasis*.

I had a blood clot a few years ago. Is that relevant to my pregnancy?
Yes. Tell your doctor about it. This is important information!

I have a blood clot in my leg, but my doctor says it isn't serious because it's 'superficial'. What does that mean?
If a blood clot occurs in the veins near the surface of the leg, it is called superficial and is not serious. This type of thrombosis does not require hospital admission and is treated with mild pain relievers, elevation of the leg, heat and support of the leg with support tights.

I have a deep vein thrombosis, and my doctor says it is a serious problem. Why?
This type of thrombosis is more serious because of the risk of the blood clot breaking loose and travelling to another part of the body, such as

the lungs. This is called a *pulmonary embolus*.

What are the signs and symptoms of a deep vein thrombosis?
Signs and symptoms of a deep vein thrombosis can vary widely and include:

- paleness of the leg
- leg is cool to the touch
- a portion of the leg may be tender, hot and swollen
- skin of the leg may have red steaks over the veins
- squeezing the calf or walking may be very painful
- rapid, abrupt onset of the above symptoms

How is a deep vein thrombosis diagnosed?
In a pregnant woman, an ultrasound scan of the legs is the only test that is done. In a non-pregnant person, either X-ray or ultrasound is used.

How is deep vein thrombosis treated during pregnancy?
Treatment usually consists of hospital admission and the administering of heparin to thin the blood and allow the clot to be dissolved. While heparin is being given, the woman is sometimes required to stay in bed with her leg elevated.

I had a blood clot with my last pregnancy and have just found out I'm pregnant. What should I do?
Call your doctor. If you had a blood clot with a previous pregnancy, you may need heparin during this one.

If heparin is to be given to prevent another blood clot, how is it given?
This is done either by injections that you give yourself 2 or 3 times a day, with an intravenous infusion or with a heparin pump.

Isn't there a blood thinner that can be taken as a pill?
Yes, it is called *warfarin*, but it is not usually given during pregnancy because it is not safe for the baby. Heparin is safe for use during pregnancy. After you deliver, you may have to take warfarin for a few weeks, depending on the severity of the blood clot.

How common is a pulmonary embolism in pregnancy?
It is an uncommon problem in pregnancy and occurs only once in every 3,000 to 7,000 deliveries.

Breast Lumps in Pregnancy

I'm pregnant and have just found a lump in my breast. What should I do?
Tell your doctor immediately! It's normal for your breasts to change and get larger during pregnancy, but lumps need to be checked out.

Are there any tests that can be done if I am pregnant and have a breast lump?
The first test is to examine yourself, then if you find a lump have your doctor check it. After examination by your doctor, either a mammogram or an ultrasound scan may be done. If a mammogram is done, be sure to tell them you are pregnant. They will cover your abdomen with a lead shield.

What can be done for a breast lump during pregnancy?
Often a lump in the breast can be drained or aspirated. If it cannot be drained, biopsy or removal of the lump may be necessary. Depending on how serious it is, surgery or other treatment may be needed.

Does a breast lump always mean cancer?
No, it doesn't, but it is very important to get breast lumps checked.

Does pregnancy make a breast cancer grow faster?
Not everyone agrees on the answer to this question. Most medical experts don't believe pregnancy accelerates the course or growth of a breast cancer.

Toxaemia of Pregnancy

I've heard about toxaemia of pregnancy. What is it?
Toxaemia of pregnancy, also called *pre-eclampsia*, is development of the following symptoms:

- hypertension (high blood pressure)
- protein in the urine

- swelling, usually in the legs, or elsewhere in the body
- changes in muscle reflexes

Toxaemia develops in about 5 per cent of pregnancies, usually in a woman's first pregnancy.

Why is toxaemia serious during pregnancy?

Toxaemia occurs only during pregnancy. It is serious because it can lead to eclampsia.

What is eclampsia?

Eclampsia refers to seizures or convulsions in a woman with toxaemia (pre-eclampsia).

What is a seizure?

A *seizure* is a loss of body control, as when someone passes out. Seizures often include twitching, shaking or convulsions of the body. If you think you've had a seizure, contact your doctor immediately!

How can I know if my toxaemia is getting worse and I am beginning to develop eclampsia?

Warning signs that toxaemia is getting worse include:

- pain under the ribs on the right side
- headache
- seeing spots or other changes in your vision

If my legs are swollen, does it mean I have toxaemia?

No, it does not. Most pregnant women experience some swelling in various parts of the body. Development of toxaemia includes evidence of the other symptoms in addition to swelling.

Does an elevation in my blood pressure mean I am getting toxaemia?

Again, you may experience some of the effects without having protein in the urine or ankle swelling.

What causes toxaemia?

Researchers have not been able to isolate a definite cause for toxaemia, but it occurs most often during a woman's first pregnancy.

How is toxaemia treated?
The goal in treating toxaemia is to avoid seizures, which occur if the woman develops eclampsia. To treat toxaemia, the first step is bed rest. The woman is also advised to drink lots of water, and avoid salt and foods containing large amounts of sodium.

If toxaemia doesn't get better with bed rest, drinking fluids and avoiding salt and sodium, then what?
In some cases, medication is prescribed to prevent seizures. The drugs used include magnesium sulphate or anti-seizure medicines, such as phenobarbitone, and drugs that reduce blood pressure.

When Your Water Breaks

I've heard about my 'water breaking'. What does this mean?
When your water breaks, the amniotic sac which surrounds the baby and placenta actually ruptures. The amniotic fluid inside the sac may gush out, then leak out more slowly. This occurrence often signals the beginning of labour.

What is the 'bag of waters'?
This is another name for the amniotic sac.

Every once in a while I feel a little wetness – as though I'm losing urine. Why does this happen?
As your pregnancy grows, your uterus grows larger and gets heavier. The uterus sits on top of the bladder – as it increases in size, it can put a great deal of pressure on your bladder and prevent it from holding as much as it did before. Leakages can occur, especially when you lift something or bounce up and down. You may notice that your underwear or clothing is damp.

How do I know my water isn't broken when I find my clothing wet?
It may be very difficult to tell the difference between losing a little urine and your water breaking. However, when your membranes rupture, you usually experience a gush of fluid or a continual leaking from inside the vagina. If you think your water has broken, call your doctor.

What does amniotic fluid look like?
It is usually clear, but it may have a bloody appearance or it may be yellow or green.

What should I do when my water breaks?
If you think your water has broken, call your doctor or midwife. Don't have sexual intercourse if you think your water has broken; it can increase the possibility of an infection inside your uterus.

Are there any tests that can be done to determine if my water has broken?
Yes, there are. One is a *nitrazine test*. Fluid is placed on a piece of nitrazine paper; if membranes have ruptured, the paper changes colour. Another test is a *ferning test*. When viewed under a microscope, dried amniotic fluid looks like a fern or the branches of a pine tree.

Problems with the Placenta

I've heard of a woman having problems with the placenta. What is the placenta?
The placenta is a flat, spongy structure that grows inside the mother's uterus. It is attached to the fetus by the umbilical cord and carries nourishment and oxygen from the mother to the baby. It also carries waste products from the baby to the mother for excretion.

I have a friend who had placenta praevia. What is this?
With *placenta praevia*, the placenta covers part or all of the cervix.

Why is this a problem?
It's a problem because when the cervix begins to dilate (open) the placenta is pulled away from the uterus, causing heavy bleeding. This can be dangerous for the mother-to-be and the baby.

What are the signs and symptoms of placenta praevia?
The most characteristic symptom in placenta praevia is painless bleeding.

If I experience this painless bleeding, what will my doctor do?
If you doctor is concerned about placenta praevia, he or she will order an ultrasound scan to determine the location of the placenta. Your

physician will *not* do a pelvic examination if he or she is concerned about placenta praevia because it may cause heavier bleeding. If you see another doctor or when you go to the hospital, tell whoever examines you that you have placenta praevia and should not have a pelvic examination.

Are there things I shouldn't do if I know I have placenta praevia?
Most physicians recommend avoiding intercourse, not travelling and not having a pelvic examination.

If I have placenta praevia, will I have to have a caesarean section?
With placenta praevia, the baby is more likely to be in a breech position. For this reason, and also to avoid bleeding, a caesarean section is almost always performed.

How common is placenta praevia?
It occurs in about 1 birth in 200.

In an article about pregnancy problems, I read about placental abruption being very serious. Can you explain what it is?
Placental abruption is separation of the placenta from the wall of the uterus during pregnancy. Normally the placenta does not separate until after delivery of the baby.

Is placental abruption dangerous?
When the placenta separates before birth, it can be very serious for the baby, and even cause fetal death.

How often does it occur?
The frequency of placental abruption is estimated to be about 1 in every 80 deliveries.

What causes placental abruption?
The cause of placental abruption is unknown; however, certain conditions may make it more likely to occur. These include:

- trauma to the mother, such as from a fall or a car accident
- an umbilical cord that is too short
- very sudden change in the size of the uterus, such as with the rupture of membranes
- hypertension (high blood pressure)

- dietary deficiency
- an abnormality of the uterus, such as a band of tissue in the uterus called a *uterine septum*

How will I know if I have placental abruption?
The signs and symptoms of placental abruption include:

- heavy bleeding from the vagina
- uterine tenderness
- uterine contractions
- premature labour
- lower back pain

Placental abruption may occur without the presence of any or all these symptoms.

Are there any tests available to help diagnose placental abruption?
Ultrasound scanning may be helpful, but it does not always provide an exact diagnosis.

What are the risks to the mother-to-be with placental abruption?
Risks to the mother-to-be include shock, severe blood loss and the inability of the blood to clot.

How is it treated?
The most common treatment of placental abruption is delivery of the baby. However, the decision about when to deliver the baby varies, depending on the severity of the problem.

If I have placental abruption, does it mean I have to have a caesarean section?
In some situations, if the baby needs to be delivered rapidly, you will need a caesarean section. But each case *must* be handled on an individual basis.

Can a woman do anything to prevent placental abruption?
Some doctors believe deficiency of folic acid may play a role in causing placental abruption. Extra folic acid may be prescribed during pregnancy. Smoking and drinking alcohol may make it more likely for a woman to have placental abruption. If you smoke or drink alcohol, you may be advised to stop both activities.

I've heard about something called a 'retained placenta'. What is this?

One complication following the birth of a baby is an abnormally adherent placenta, which means a placenta that does not deliver following the birth of the baby. This is called a *retained placenta*. Usually the placenta separates on its own from the implantation site on the uterus a few minutes after delivery. In some cases, it doesn't separate because it is attached to the wall of the uterus. This can be very serious and can cause extreme blood loss.

What causes a retained placenta?

Some reasons for a retained placenta include a placenta attaching:

• over a previous caesarean section scar or other incision scar on the uterus
• in a place that has been curetted (scraped), such as with a D and C
• over an area of the uterus that was infected

What kind of problems does a retained placenta cause?

The most significant problem is heavy bleeding after delivery. If the placenta is not delivered, it must be removed some other way. One solution is to perform a D and C. However, if the placenta has grown into the wall of the uterus, occasionally it may be necessary to remove the uterus by performing a hysterectomy.

Is a retained placenta common?

No. It occurs in about 1 per cent of all deliveries.

CHAPTER 16

You should also Know

How does the doctor determine my due date?
You due date is set at 38 weeks after the date the baby was conceived. If you don't know the exact date of conception, it is estimated to be near the middle of your menstrual cycle, or two weeks after the beginning of your last period. Once your doctor knows the date of conception, he counts 38 weeks from that date to determine your due date.

Another way to estimate the date of delivery is to take the date of the beginning of your last period, add 7 days and go back 3 months. Both methods give the same result.

I get confused by the terms 'gestational age' and 'fertilisation age'. Why are two ages used?
Gestational age is the length of time since the beginning of your last period. If you doctor says you are 15 weeks pregnant, he or she is referring to your gestational age. *Fertilisation age* is the actual age of the fetus, which would be 13 weeks in this case.

What about 'trimesters'? My sister told me there are three trimesters during pregnancy.
That's correct. *Trimesters* divide pregnancy into three stages, each about 13 weeks long. It helps group together times of development.

I'm 13 weeks pregnant, but I don't show yet and don't feel very pregnant. How do I know everything is all right?
At this point, a lot has happened with the development of your baby. There are a few outward signs that can help reassure you. If you have seen your doctor in the last couple of weeks, you have probably heard

the baby's heart beat. In the middle of your abdomen just above your pubic bone you may feel your uterus, which will feel like the top of a smooth ball, about the size of a large grapefruit.

Some Common Physical Concerns

My feet are huge – I can't wear any of my shoes. What can I do about it?
Some swelling in your feet is normal during pregnancy. Wear trainers, flats or shoes with low heels (no higher than 2in/5cm). If swelling becomes extreme, especially during the last trimester, consult your physician; it could be a sign of problems. Rest lying down on your side as frequently as possible. You may need to buy larger shoes towards the end of your pregnancy.

What is sciatic nerve pain?
Sciatic nerve pain is an occasional excruciating pain in your buttocks and down the back or the side of your leg. You may experience it as your pregnancy progresses. The sciatic nerve runs behind the uterus in the pelvis to your legs. Pain is believed to be caused by pressure on the nerve from the growing uterus.

What can I do about sciatic nerve pain?
The best way to treat the pain is to lie on your opposite side. It helps relieve pressure on the nerve.

I've heard that backaches are a normal part of pregnancy. What causes them?
Nearly every woman experiences backache at some time during her pregnancy. It usually occurs as you get bigger. You may also experience backache after walking, bending, lifting, standing or excessive exercise. Be careful about lifting and bending – do it correctly.

How do I take care of problems with my back?
You can treat backache with heat, rest and analgesics, such as paracetamol (Panadol). Special maternity girdles can provide some support. Keep your weight under control, and take some mild exercise, such as swimming, walking and stationary-bike riding. Try to lie on your side when resting or sleeping.

Should I be concerned about lower back pain?
Lower back pain is common during pregnancy. However it may be an indication of a more serious problem, such as pyelonephritis or a kidney stone. If pain becomes constant or more severe, it's important to discuss it with your doctor.

I've heard that lying on my side in the third trimester will help with any swelling I have. Is this true?
Yes, it is. By the third trimester, your uterus is quite large and puts a lot of pressure on your blood vessels, blocking their flow. Lying or sleeping or your side during the third trimester will help relieve this.

The Emotions of Pregnancy

Now that I know I'm pregnant, I'm not as excited as I thought I'd be. Is this normal?
If you aren't immediately thrilled about pregnancy, don't feel alone. A very common feeling or response to pregnancy is to question your condition. Some of this may be because you're not sure of what lies ahead.

When will I begin to think of the fetus as my 'baby'?
This is different for everyone. Some women begin to feel this way as soon as they know they are pregnant. For others, it occurs when they hear their baby's heart beat, around 12 or 13 weeks, or when they first feel their baby move, between 16 and 20 weeks.

I'm not very far along in my pregnancy, but I seem to be very emotional about everything. Is this normal?
Yes, it's perfectly normal to get very emotional about many things. You may feel moody, cry at the slightest thing or find yourself day-dreaming. Emotional swings are very normal during pregnancy.

Will these emotional swings continue during my pregnancy?
They continue to some degree throughout pregnancy. These swings are caused by the changing hormones in your body. Explain to your partner and other family members that you may experience these swings.

Your Maternity Wardrobe

Now that I know I'm pregnant, I'm excited about wearing maternity clothes. When will I need them?
It's very hard to predict exactly when you'll need to start wearing maternity clothes. You may already have some clothes that are loose enough to wear for a while. You might be able to wear some of your partner's shirts. A rule of thumb to follow is, when you become uncomfortable wearing your regular clothes, it's time to start wearing maternity clothes.

Are there any points I should keep in mind when selecting maternity clothes?
Choose natural fabrics when possible – avoid synthetics. During pregnancy, your metabolic rate increases, and you may feel warmer than usual. You'll want to wear fabrics that 'breathe'. Wear cotton in the summer, and layer your clothing in winter.

There are so many different styles of clothing for a pregnant woman. Are any styles better than others?
It depends on your preference, but I'll share with you some of the tips my patients have given me. They have found the following styles added to their comfort:

• wide, elastic bands or panels that fit under the abdomen to provide support
• wrap-around openings that tie and are easy to adjust
• elastic waists that expand
• button or pleated waistbands that are adjustable
• waistbands that have sliders to adjust the fit

My friend told me that I should wear special maternity underwear while I'm pregnant. What did she mean?
Undergarments that add support to your abdomen, breasts or legs may make you feel more comfortable during pregnancy. These undergarments include maternity bras, nursing bras, maternity knickers and maternity support tights. Be sure to choose knickers and support tights with a cotton crotch.

What are maternity bras?
Maternity bras are designed to provide your enlarging breasts with the extra support they need during pregnancy. They have wider sides and stretchier backs than your regular bras. They usually have four sets of hooks on the back, instead of two or three, providing more room for you to grow.

Can't I just wear my normal bra in a larger size?
It's probably better to buy a maternity bra. They can help combat the stretch marks and sagging of the breasts which are associated with pregnancy.

What is a nursing bra?
A nursing bra is worn for breastfeeding; it has cups that open so you can breast feed without having to undress. Buy a nursing bra *only* if you plan to breast feed your baby. You won't need one if you bottle feed.

When should I buy a nursing bra?
Wait until the final weeks of your pregnancy; don't buy one before 36 weeks. Your breasts won't be large enough to get a correct fit before then.

How can I be sure that a nursing bra will fit correctly?
Choose a nursing bra with about a finger's width of space between any part of the cup and your breast. This allows for the enlargement of your breasts when your milk comes in. For a better fit, take nursing pads with you when shopping for a nursing bra. Choose a bra that is comfortable when fastened on the loosest row of hooks (to allow for shrinkage in your rib cage after pregnancy).

What are maternity knickers?
These knickers provide support for your enlarging abdomen. Some have panels for your abdomen; others have a wide elastic band that fits under your abdomen to provide support. These knickers may be most comfortable in the last trimester of pregnancy.

Will I have to wear maternity support tights?
Many women do *not* have to wear support tights during pregnancy. However, if you have a family history of varicose veins or if you develop them during pregnancy, you may need to wear them. Don't depend on over-the-counter support tights. You'll need to visit a vein

specialist to have maternity support tights personally fitted. See Chapter 9 for additional information on varicose veins and support tights.

Can I wear regular tights?

If you don't have any problems with varicose veins, ordinary tights are all right. Choose those with a stretchy, wide, non-binding waistband, and wear them over or below your abdomen, whichever is more comfortable. You might also be able to buy maternity tights.

Choosing your Baby's Doctor

My friend told me that I should pick my baby's doctor before the baby is born. Is this true?

Yes. It's best to choose and visit your doctor *before* your baby is born. An interview will help you build a partnership for your child's health and well-being. You can talk with the doctor about the care of your baby, ask questions about feeding and receive some guidelines about dealing with a new baby.

Who will be my baby's doctor?

Usually your family doctor or one of his partners will specialise in paediatric care. Your baby may also be seen at the hospital to check that all is well, and your baby will be referred to the hospital if there is any serious problem.

I'm sure there are certain questions we should ask our doctor before the baby arrives. What are some of them?

There are many things that may worry you. Below is a list of questions that I believe will help you create a useful dialogue.

- Are your surgery hours compatible with our work schedules?
- Can an acutely ill child be seen the same day?
- How can we reach you in case of an emergency or after surgery hours?
- Who responds if you are not available?
- Do you return telephone calls?
- Are you interested in preventive, developmental and behavioural issues with babies and infants?
- What is the nearest (to our home) hospital emergency department you would send us to?

What other things should we think about when considering the doctor for our baby?
There are some issues that can be resolved only by analysing your feelings after seeing the doctor – examining your 'gut reactions' to certain issues. Below is a list of questions you and your partner might want to discuss after seeing him or her.

• Are the doctor's philosophies and attitudes acceptable to us, such as use of antibiotics and other medicines, child-rearing practices or medical-related religious beliefs?
• Did the doctor listen to us?
• Was he or she genuinely interested in our concerns?
• Did the doctor appear interested in developing a rapport with our expected child?
• Is this a person I feel comfortable with and with whom our child will be comfortable?

What if we don't like the doctor who deals with babies in our general practice?
You should consider changing to another general practice, and particularly to one where one of the partners has a specialist qualification in paediatrics. Ask your local Family Health Authority.

Travelling during Pregnancy

I've got to make a business trip soon, and I'm pregnant. Can I go?
Travel during pregnancy can be fatiguing and frustrating, but if your pregnancy is normal you should be able to travel during the first and second trimesters without too much trouble. Consult your physician if you're considering travelling during your third trimester.

What should I keep in mind about travelling while I'm pregnant?
Take frequent breaks to stretch your legs during trips. Don't overdo it – rest when possible. You might want to avoid places where good medical care is not available or where changes in climate, food or altitude could cause you problems.

Is it all right to fly?
Flying in itself should not cause you any problems. Try to get an aisle seat, so you can stretch your legs and get up to walk about more easily.

Drink plenty of fluids, such as water and juice, because the recirculated air in an aircraft is extremely dry. Discuss with your doctor any plans you have for flying. Some airlines refuse to carry a pregnant passenger without the written consent of her doctor.

I'm just finishing my first trimester, and we are planning a trip. Is this all right?
Ask your doctor. Most will tell you it's all right to travel during pregnancy, but each situation is different. Some general considerations about travelling during pregnancy include the following.

- Don't plan a trip during your last month of pregnancy.
- If you're having any problems, such as bleeding or cramping, don't travel.
- If you are uncomfortable or have problems with swelling, then travelling, sitting in a car or doing a lot of walking may make things worse (and they probably won't be much fun either).
- If your pregnancy is considered 'high risk', a trip during pregnancy is not a good idea.

Remember you are pregnant when you plan a trip. Be sensible in your planning – don't overdo it – and take it easy!

What are the greatest risks for me if I decide to travel during my pregnancy?
The biggest risk in travelling during pregnancy is the development of a complication while you are away from home and away from those who have been involved in your pregnancy and know your history. You should also think again if you are experiencing discomfort or having trouble sleeping, especially if you are going to be cooped up in a car for hours or will have to sleep in a strange bed. Consider these things and discuss them with your doctor before making plans, buying tickets or making reservations.

I've heard I shouldn't travel during the last month of my pregnancy. Why?
At this point, labour could begin at any time, your water could break or other problems could occur. You doctor knows what has happened during your pregnancy and has a record of tests done – these things are important. If you check into a hospital in a strange place, they don't know you and you don't know them. Some doctors won't accept you as a patient in this situation, and it can be awkward. It doesn't make sense to take this kind of chance.

Can't my doctor check me and tell if I will be in labour soon so I'll know if I can go on a trip?

First of all, *no one* can predict when your labour will begin. No one can therefore guarantee that you can go on a trip and not go into labour or have other problems. You can't guarantee it – even if you stay at home! So, if you're thinking of going on a trip, discuss it with your doctor *before* you make detailed plans or buy tickets.

My husband has to go out of town for a business trip, and I'm due in 3 weeks. Can't my doctor check me and tell if I will go into labour while he's gone?

If you husband goes on his trip, he may miss the delivery. Your doctor can check you, but this really only tells you where you are at *that* point in time. Nothing will *guarantee* your husband won't miss the delivery. The last month of pregnancy isn't a good time for either of you to be travelling.

Driving and Seat-belt Use in Pregnancy

Is it safe for me to drive during pregnancy?

Yes, it's safe to drive throughout your pregnancy. It may become uncomfortable for you to get in and out of the car as pregnancy progresses, but being pregnant should not interfere with your ability to drive.

I always wear a seat belt with I drive, but I'm wondering if a seat belt could cause me problems now that I'm pregnant. Should I wear one?

Yes! Many women are confused about wearing seat belts or shoulder harnesses during pregnancy, but don't be misled. These safety restraints are necessary during pregnancy, just as they are necessary when you're not pregnant.

Will wearing a safety belt hurt my baby?

There is no evidence of safety restraints increasing the chance of fetal or uterine injury. You have a better chance of survival in an accident wearing a seat belt than not wearing one.

Is there a proper way for me to wear a seat belt while I'm pregnant?
Yes. Place the lap belt part of the restraint *below* your abdomen and *across* your upper thighs so it's snug and comfortable. Adjust your sitting position so the belt crosses your shoulder without cutting into your neck. Position the shoulder harness between your breasts; don't slip this belt off your shoulder.

If I decide to have private care by an obstetrician for the pregnancy and delivery, how much is it likely to cost?
The cost will be the fees charged by the obstetrician and paediatrician and the hospital charges.

Most obstetricians give a 'package deal' for private antenatal care and delivery, and do not vary this if delivery has to be by forceps or caesarean section. In and about London, the obstetrician's fee varies from £1,000 to £2,500, but you may have to budget for as much as £750 for special antenatal tests. In areas outside London, charges may be less. You should telephone the secretary of an obstetrician in your area to enquire what his or her charges are. Your family doctor will know which obstetricians provide private care. Hospital charges for a normal delivery and stay of 2 to 3 days are £1,500 to £2,500 in London, but if you have an operative vaginal delivery by forceps or a caesarean section you may have to pay up to £1,000 to £1,500 more. Again, provincial hospitals may charge less, and you should check by telephone with the Private Patients Department at your local hospital, or with a nearby private maternity hospital. Your family doctor will be able to advise on which hospitals provide a private service. There may be an additional charge of up to £50 per day for the care of the newborn baby.

If you want to select a private paediatrician you will have to check with his or her secretary to find out his or her daily fee. The care your baby will get will not be very different from that provided by the hospital paediatrician.

What will it cost if I have a premature baby needing intensive care?
A very premature baby may have to stay in hospital as long as 3 months and the cost of private care could be very great, between £5,000 and £20,000. The care your premature baby will have will not differ significantly from that provided under the National Health Service, which in general makes no charges, and you would be wise to consider this alternative.

I have private health insurance. Will this cover the cost of private care for the pregnancy and delivery?
This varies according to the health insurance company, and according to the policy you have. You must check with the insurance company. Some policies do not cover any costs related to pregnancies. Some major health insurers will only pay for an evacuation of the uterus after a miscarriage or an emergency caesarean section. Some have policies which cover all complications of pregnancy and delivery, but policies which cope with the expenses of a normal pregnancy and delivery are hard to find.

Antenatal Classes

When should I register for antenatal classes?
Plan ahead. When you are around 20 weeks pregnant, begin looking into classes that are offered at your hospital or elsewhere in your area. You should be signed up or just starting classes by the beginning of the third trimester or about 27 weeks. It's a good idea to plan to finish the classes at least a few weeks before you are due.

Why should I take antenatal classes?
Classes are a good way to prepare for a very important and exciting time in your life! You will also benefit from mixing with other people who have the same concerns as you.

Where are antenatal classes held?
Childbirth classes are offered in various places. Most hospitals that deliver babies offer antenatal classes at the hospital. They are often taught by midwives. Ask your doctor about which classes would be best for you.

Are antenatal classes only for first-time mothers?
No. Classes are recommended for first-time pregnant women, women with a new partner, if it has been a few years since you've had a baby, if you have questions or if you would like a review of labour and delivery.

I want to take some childbirth education classes to prepare me for my baby's birth. How do I find them?

First, ask your doctor to recommend classes in your area. He or she is familiar with what is being offered. Check local hospitals; many offer these classes. Friends can also be good sources. The National Childbirth Trust (tel 0181 992 8637) has branches throughout the country and runs antenatal classes.

Do many couples take childbirth education classes?

Yes. Most first-time expectant parents take some type of childbirth education class.

Do these classes really help?

They seem to. Some studies suggest that women who have taken classes need less medication, have fewer forceps deliveries and feel more positive about the birth than women who do not take classes.

What kind of things will we learn about in childbirth classes?

Classes cover many aspects of labour and delivery, including breathing techniques, vaginal birth, caesarean section, hospital procedures, ways to deal with the discomfort and pain of labour and delivery, various pain-relief methods and the post-natal or recovery period.

What are Lamaze classes?

Lamaze is the oldest technique of childbirth preparation. It emphasises relaxation and breathing as ways to relax during labour and delivery.

How will I know a class is right for me?

There are quite a few things you can do.

- Find out what is available in your area.
- Talk to friends and relatives who have taken various classes.
- Decide whether you want a drug-free birth or whether you are willing to consider pain relief if it is necessary.
- Learn about the qualifications of the instructors in various programmes.
- Visit some classes in your area to choose the best one for you.

Other Pregnancy Questions

I have a couple of friends who got pregnant at about the same time as I did, but we all look as if we're at different stages of pregnancy. Is there anything wrong?

Probably not. Everyone's pregnancy is different, and every woman reacts to pregnancy differently. A lot of what you look like depends on your size (how tall are you, your weight) and the size of your growing baby. Don't expect to look the same as other women or to have the same experience as your friends.

Is it all right to have sexual relations while I am pregnant? My partner and I don't want to do anything that would be dangerous to our baby.

For most couples it's all right to have sexual relations during pregnancy. If you're having any problems with bleeding, cramping or later in your pregnancy you think your water has broken, then it's best not to have relations. For more information on this subject, see Chapter 10.

I don't usually use sunscreen, but a friend suggested it's important during pregnancy. Why?

The use of sunscreen on your face is very important during pregnancy. It lessens the likelihood of getting the 'mask of pregnancy', which is a darkening of skin pigment on cheeks, forehead and chin. Use products with a protection factor of 15 or higher. If you are prone to acne breakouts, use a water-based or oil-free product.

How safe is it for me to have a bath during pregnancy?

Most doctors believe it is safe to have a bath during pregnancy. The only precaution is to avoid slipping and falling as you get into or out of the bath.

Someone said I shouldn't have a bath during pregnancy, that it's better to shower. Is this true?

There is no medical reason to choose showering over bathing during pregnancy. In the last few weeks of pregnancy, as you get bigger, you must be careful about slipping and falling in the shower or bath. If you think your water has broken (ruptured membranes), your doctor may recommend that you don't bath.

I've always heard that a pregnant woman shouldn't have her hair coloured or get a permanent wave. Is there any real reason to avoid these?

I don't think these should be problems for you. However, it's probably a good idea to avoid these activities during the first trimester, especially if you have morning sickness. The fumes from the hair dye or the permanent solution could make you feel ill.

I love to have a massage because it relaxes me so much. Can I continue to have massages while I'm pregnant?

It's probably all right to have a massage during pregnancy. You may find it more difficult as your pregnancy progresses and you get bigger. If you want to have a massage when you are further along in your pregnancy, lie on your side instead of on your stomach. Always be careful not to get overheated in any activity.

My breasts are really sore. Is this normal?

Changes in your breasts can begin early in your pregnancy; it isn't unusual for them to tingle or be sore. You may also notice your breasts getting larger, or see a darkening areola or an elevation of the glands around the nipple.

It seems I am always in the bathroom urinating since I became pregnant. Is this normal?

More frequent urination is common in pregnancy. Watch for signs of a urinary tract infection, such as blood in your urine, a fever or burning or pain when your urinate.

We have a dog that has been our 'baby' for 6 years. Now we are expecting a real baby. Will we have problems with our pet?

When a baby is born to a couple with a dog that has been the centre of attention for a long while, problems may arise. Sometimes the dog resents the attention the baby gets and growls at the infant, barks or demands attention. The animal may even revert to unacceptable behaviour, such as wetting or tearing things up.

What can we do to help our pet accept the new baby?

If you dog has never been used to children, begin introducing it to the sights, sounds and smells of a new baby before yours is born. Put the baby's crib in place weeks in advance. When you bring the baby home, give your dog positive attention while introducing it to the new baby.

Be firm when your dog misbehaves – don't let it get away with bad behaviour. Unneutered dogs may be more apt to growl, snap and bite. Don't isolate your dog when you bring the baby home. Try to involve the dog in some of your routines with the baby. Don't leave the dog alone with the baby. Use common sense, and take things slowly.

We have a cat. Should we expect problems with it when we bring the baby home?
Cats are affected in many of the same ways as dogs, and much of the advice on dogs applies to cats. Expect a cat to take longer to adjust to a new baby than a dog does. You will have to train your cat to stay out of the baby's cot.

We've been considering names for our baby; some of them are unusual. Should we discuss our choices with others?
I have one patient who told me she and her husband decide on a name together, but don't tell anyone else until after the baby is born. She said it's very easy for people to criticise a name when you're thinking about it, but few people will tell you they don't like a name when you've already given it to your baby!

Is it all right to use the microwave during my pregnancy?
We don't know for sure if there is danger to your pregnancy from using a microwave oven, so follow the directions in the manual carefully. It's a good idea not to stand next to or directly in front of it while it's in use.

Would it be all right to take my partner with me to my appointments with the doctor?
It's a great idea! It will help him realise what is happening to you and to feel a part of your pregnancy. And it's nice for your partner and your doctor and midwife to meet before labour begins.

Can I take anyone else with me to my appointments?
It's all right to take your mother or mother-in-law with you to an appointment to hear the baby's heart beat. Things have really changed since your mother carried you; she might enjoy this type of visit. If you want to bring anyone else, discuss if first with your doctor or midwife.

My children are curious and ask a lot of questions about my pregnancy. Is it all right to take them with me to my antenatal appointments?

Many clinics don't mind if you bring your children with you; others ask you not to bring children along. Ask about the clinic's policy. If you're having problems and need to talk to your doctor, it can be very difficult to do this if you're also trying to take care of a young child.

Do you have any suggestions for me if I do bring my children with me?

Some suggestions for bringing children including the following.

- Ask about the clinic's policy ahead of time.
- Don't bring them on your first visit, when you will probably have a pelvic examination.
- If you're bringing your children to hear the heart beat, don't bring them the first time your doctor tries to hear it; wait until after you have heard it first.
- Bring one child at a time rather than a large group.
- Bring something to 'entertain' your child in case you have to wait – not all clinics have toys or books for children.
- Be considerate of other patients; don't bring a child who has a cold or is sick. I've had patients bring their children with them then tell me the child had chicken pox or a sore throat! This could be very serious for other pregnant women sitting in the waiting room.

I've been hearing about how important the placenta is during pregnancy. Can you tell me more about it?

The placenta, which attaches to the umbilical cord of the baby, transports oxygen to the baby and carries away carbon dioxide. It is involved in the baby's nutrition and the baby's excretion of waste products. It also plays a very important role in hormone production during pregnancy.

Does the placenta protect my baby?

The placenta acts as a filter for many substances passing from you to your baby, including certain drugs and infections that can't pass through the placenta to the baby.

I'm confused about the placenta and the birth of my baby. Is the placenta delivered separately?

Yes. Stage 3 of labour involves the delivery of the placenta. After the birth of your baby, the uterus contracts and expels the placenta. Once the placenta has been delivered, the birth process is complete. For further information, see Chapter 17.

Some Pregnancy Warnings

I like to sit in a Jacuzzi after I exercise, but I have read that I shouldn't while I'm pregnant. Why?

Your baby relies on you to maintain the correct body temperature. Research has shown that an elevated temperature lasting several minutes many harm a developing fetus, so for this reason it's best to avoid Jacuzzi, saunas, steamrooms and spas during pregnancy.

I like to look tanned all year long, so I use a sunbed. This won't harm my baby, will it?

Researchers have not studied the effects on a growing fetus when a pregnant woman lies on a sunbed. Until we know that there is no reason for concern, don't do this while you're pregnant.

Is it all right to douche during pregnancy?

No. Most doctors agree douching can be dangerous during pregnancy.

What's the problem with douching during pregnancy?

Using a douche may cause an infection or bleeding or even break your bag of waters (rupture your membranes). It can cause more serious problems, such as an *air embolus*. This occurs when air gets into your circulation from the pressure of the douche. It is rare but can be a serious problem.

I usually have electrolysis for some facial hair I have. Can I have this done during pregnancy?

No one knows for sure whether this procedure is safe or not. Because there is no information available, I would suggest you wait until after your baby is born to have your facial hair removed.

To remove leg hair, I have my legs waxed. Is this permissible while I'm pregnant?

I don't believe there is any risk to you with this procedure. Just be sure you don't get overheated while having it done. You shouldn't raise your body temperature above 100.6°F (38°C) for more than 15 minutes.

When I was 15 I had my shoulder tattooed, but I want to have it removed now. My dermatologist told me to wait till after the baby is born. Why?

Many tattoos are removed using lasers, and we are unsure how safe it might be for you to have this done during pregnancy. I agree with your dermatologist – wait until after your baby is born to have it removed.

I have just received a gift token for a herbal wrap, and I'm 14 weeks pregnant. Should I wait until after my baby is born?

Definitely wait until after your baby is born to have a herbal wrap. Being wrapped in hot towels will cause your body to become very heated, which is not advisable during pregnancy.

Can I continue to use my electric blanket now that I'm pregnant?

There has been controversy about using electric blankets during pregnancy. At this time, no one knows the answer to this question. Until we know more, the safest thing to do is not to use an electric blanket but to find other ways to stay warm, such as with down comforters or extra blankets.

Everybody at work seems to have advice for me. How do I handle this?

Unwelcome advice, unwarranted questions, even physical contact are common during pregnancy. Use humour to deflect some of the questions. You can listen to unasked-for advice, nod wisely and say 'thanks', without making any commitment. Try not to let this attention annoy you.

I find it annoying when people (even total strangers) pat my pregnant abdomen. How can I stop them or keep them from doing this?

You can ask people to look and not touch! When someone reaches out to touch your abdomen, tell them you don't like people doing that.

Down's Syndrome

What is Down's syndrome?

Down's syndrome is a condition in which a baby is born mentally retarded and often physically deformed. His or her appearance may include a sloping forehead, short, broad hands, a flat nose and low-set ears. There may also be heart problems, gastrointestinal defects or leukaemia. Down's syndrome is caused by a defective chromosome.

Can Down's syndrome be diagnosed before the baby is born?

Yes. Traditionally amniocentesis has been used to diagnose Down's syndrome. Other tests that may prove useful include alpha-fetoprotein, chorionic villus sampling and, in some cases, ultrasound scanning. For further information on Down's syndrome, see Chapter 3.

PART **III**

The Birth of your Baby

CHAPTER 17

Labour and Delivery

**I've already felt some contractions, and I'm only 6 months pregnant.
Am I going into labour?**
Probably not. You are probably experiencing Braxton-Hicks
contractions, which are painless, non-rhythmical contractions. They
can begin early in pregnancy and continue off and on until your baby
is born. They are felt at irregular intervals and may increase in number
and strength when your uterus is massaged.

**I heard a woman describe her baby as 'dropping'. Does this mean
the baby was falling out?**
No, it doesn't. The feeling of having your baby drop, also called
lightening, means the baby's head has moved down deep into your
pelvis. It is a natural part of the birthing process and can happen a few
weeks to a few hours before labour begins.

Will I feel better when my baby drops?
You may feel that you have more room to breathe when the baby
descends into your pelvis, but there may also be more pelvic pressure
or discomfort.

**I've heard horror stories about a woman's water breaking when she
was out in public. Does this happen often?**
Many mothers-to-be worry about the embarrassment of having their
bag of waters break when they are in a public place. Although it
doesn't happen very often, it is possible. Don't waste energy worrying
about it. If it should happen to you, people are likely to be very
understanding and helpful. At that stage of your pregnancy, your
condition would be very obvious to them!

Does the water usually break before a woman goes into labour?

Many times the water will break shortly before labour begins. However, in most cases the doctor must rupture the membranes after the woman goes to the hospital.

How will I know when my water breaks?

Your baby is surrounded by *amniotic fluid* in the uterus. Often, as labour begins, the membranes that surround the baby break and fluid leaks from your vagina. You may feel a gush of fluid, followed by slow leaking, or you may feel just a slow leaking without the gush of fluid. A sanitary pad will help absorb the slow leaking so you are not embarrassed by it.

What should I do when my water breaks?

Contact your doctor or midwife immediately; some precautions must be taken. If labour and delivery are imminent, you may be advised to go to the hospital. If you are not near term, your doctor may ask you to come to his surgery, where you will be examined. You may not be ready to deliver your baby yet, and your doctor wants to prevent you getting an infection. The risk of infection increases when your water breaks.

My doctor said she might have to induce me. How is this done?

If labour is induced, your bag of waters will be broken or you will receive oxytocin (Syntocinon) intravenously. The drug is given in gradually increasing doses until contractions begin.

Why is labour induced?

Your doctor may decide to induce labour if you or your baby is at risk, for example if you are overdue. If the cervix is dilated and contractions have not begun or are not strong enough, your labour may be induced.

Is there any way for my doctor to know when I will go into labour?

No one knows when labour will begin.

How long does labour last?

The length of your labour is extremely individual. It varies from pregnancy to pregnancy and depends on how many pregnancies you have already had.

How long can I expect to be in labour with a first baby?
With a first pregnancy, the first and second stages of labour can last 14 to 15 hours, or more. A woman who had already had one or two children will probably have a shorter labour, but that's not always the case.

Premature Labour

What is 'preterm birth'?
Preterm birth refers to a baby born more than 4 weeks early. It is also called *premature birth.*

How common is preterm birth?
About 10 per cent of all babies are born more than 4 weeks early.

I've heard preterm birth can be dangerous for the baby. Why?
Preterm delivery of a baby can be dangerous because the baby's lungs and other organ systems may not be ready to function on their own.

What causes premature labour?
In most cases, the cause of premature labour is unknown. Causes we do understand include:

• a uterus with an abnormal shape
• a large uterus (such as with twin pregnancies)
• hydramnios (excessive amniotic fluid)
• an abnormal placenta
• premature rupture of the membranes
• incompetent cervix (a weak cervix which dilates early)
• abnormalities of the fetus
• fetal death
• retained intra-uterine contraceptive device
• maternal illness, such as high blood pressure, or some maternal infections
• incorrect estimate of gestational age, which means the baby is really *not* premature

What will my doctor tell me to do if I go into labour too early?
It is important to try to halt the contractions if you go into labour too early. Most doctors start by recommending bed rest to stop labour. Bed

rest means lying in bed on your side. Either side is all right, but the left side is better.

Why do I have to lie in bed?
It works. It may mean you have to modify or stop your activities, but we have found that bed rest helps end premature labour. Before we had drugs for this, bed rest was the only treatment for premature labour. It is still often successful in halting premature labour.

I've heard there are drugs to stop premature labour. Can't I take one of those drugs instead of going to bed?
Even if you take drugs, you will probably be advised to rest in bed. Bed rest is an essential part of the treatment plan for premature labour.

What kinds of drug are used to treat premature labour?
There are two types that relax the uterus and decrease contractions:

• beta-sympathomimetics, including ritodrine and terbutaline, which are given intravenously or by injection.
• sedatives or narcotics, which may be used in early attempts to stop premature labour.

What are the benefits of stopping premature labour?
It is better for both mother and baby if premature labour is stopped. Premature delivery increases the risks of fetal problems and maternal problems, such as an increased risk of caesarean section.

Going to the Hospital

I'm nervous about preparing to go to the hospital. What should I be concerned about?
Going to the hospital to have a baby can cause anyone a little nervousness, even an experienced mother. If you make some plans before you have to go, you'll have less to worry about.

• Ask to tour the labour and delivery area of your hospital.
• Plan the trip; know who will take you, and have a backup person available.
• Make a personal plan.
• Pack your bag.

I've never had a baby before. What do I need to take with me to the hospital?
There are a lot of things to consider, but the list below should cover most of what you might need:

- 1 cotton nightgown or T-shirt for labour
- light diversion, such as books or magazines, to use during labour
- 1 nightgown for after delivery (bring a nursing gown if you are going to breast feed)
- slippers with rubber soles
- 1 long robe for walking in the corridors
- 2 bras (nursing bras and pads if you breast feed)
- toiletries you use, including brush, comb, toothbrush, toothpaste, soap, shampoo, conditioner
- hairband or hair tie, if you have long hair
- glasses (you won't be able to wear contact lenses)
- underwear and loose-fitting clothes for going home
- sanitary pads, if the hospital doesn't supply them

Should I bring anything to the hospital for my partner?
It's a good idea to include some things in your hospital kit for your partner to help him get through the experience. You might consider the following items:

- talc or oil for massaging you during labour
- a paint roller or tennis ball for giving you a low back massage during labour
- tapes or CDs and a player, or a radio to play during labour
- camera and film
- list of telephone numbers and a telephone card
- change for telephones and vending machines

What should I bring for my new baby?
The hospital will probably supply most of what you will need for your baby; however, there are a few things you should have ready:

- clothes for the trip home, including a vest, a sleeping gown and outer clothes (a hat if it's cold)
- a couple of blankets
- nappies if your hospital doesn't supply them

Be sure you have an approved infant car seat to take your baby home.

It's important to start your baby in a car seat the very first time he or she rides in a car!

If I am in labour, what can I expect once I get to the hospital?

After you are admitted, you will probably be settled into a labour room, and you will be checked to see how much you have dilated. A brief history of your pregnancy will be taken. Vital signs, including blood pressure, pulse and temperature, are noted. You may receive an enema, or intravenous fluid may be given. Blood will probably be drawn. You may have an epidural put in place, if you have requested it.

Does a woman always need to have her pubic hair shaved before the birth of her baby?

No. Most are not shaved these days. However, some patients who chose *not* to have their pubic hair shaved told me later they experienced discomfort when their pubic hair became entangled in their underwear due to the normal vaginal discharge after the birth of their baby.

Is an intravenous drip always necessary?

Intravenous fluid is necessary with an epidural. However if you have chosen not to have an epidural, it is not always required. Most physicians agree an intravenous infusion is helpful if the woman needs medication or fluids during labour.

Can I refuse to have an intravenous drip?

Discuss this with your doctor before the birth of your baby. In some situations, an intravenous infusion can save your life.

A friend told me that when she got to the hospital, she found that the midwife or doctor she had seen at the clinic was on vacation and someone she didn't know was going to deliver her baby. Is there anything I can do to prevent this from happening to me?

Talk to your doctor or midwife about this possibility. If they believe they might be away when your baby is born, ask to meet those who 'cover' when your doctor and midwife are unavailable. Although they would like to be there for the birth of your baby, sometimes it is not possible.

Labour

What does labour feel like?
Your entire abdomen (the uterus) contracts (tightens) like a hard muscle then relaxes. The tightening of the uterus can cause pain.

I've heard friends describe labour differently. One said her back hurt, another said it felt like the pain she had with diarrhoea. Are these different types of labour?
No, these are not different types of labour. Labour is different for every woman; that's the reason we can't predict what your labour will be like before it begins. You may also find you labour differently from one pregnancy to the next.

I've heard all sorts of stories about labour, but I don't really know what it is. Can you explain it for me?
Labour is defined by the *dilatation* (stretching and expanding) of your cervix. This occurs when your uterus, which is a muscle, tightens (contracts) to squeeze out its contents (your baby).

True Labour or False Labour?

Considerations	True Labour	False Labour
Contractions	Regular	Irregular
Time between contractions	Come closer together	Do not get closer together
Contraction intensity	Increases	Doesn't change
Location of contractions	Entire abdomen or back	Various locations
Effect of anaesthetic or pain relievers	Will not stop labour	Sedation may alter frequency or stop contractions
Cervical change	Progressive cervical change (effacement and dilatation)	No cervical change

How will I know the difference between true labour and false labour?

There *are* differences between the two. The chart on the previous page highlights the principal ones.

I've heard about different stages of labour. What are they?

Labour is divided into three stages – each is distinctly different and has a specific purpose. Review the chart on pages 223–4 to see what you might expect during the various stages of labour and delivery.

What is the first stage of labour?

Stage 1 of labour is the longest and consists of three phases – early, active and transition. This first stage of labour usually lasts 6 to 8 hours but can be longer for a first birth.

In the early phase, labour is just getting started and dilatation of the cervix has just begun. In the active phase, the cervix dilates at a fairly constant rate; transition includes complete dilatation. Contractions help the cervix dilate and thin out. They also help move the baby down the birth canal for delivery.

At the transition phase, the pace and intensity of labour increases, signalling that labour is moving into the second stage.

What is the second stage of labour?

In *stage 2 of labour*, your cervix is fully dilated and you begin to push. Contractions change and become much harder, longer and more frequent. Along with your pushing, these contractions help deliver the baby. This stage can take 2 hours or longer. Anaesthesia at this point, especially an epidural block, may prolong this stage of labour because your urge to push is decreased. At the end of the second stage, your baby is born.

What is the third stage of labour?

Stage 3 of labour usually takes only a few minutes. During stage 3, the uterus contracts and expels the placenta (after-birth). You may be given an injection of Syntometrine (oxytocin with ergometrine) or oxytocin alone to help the uterus contract.

Somewhere I read there's a fourth stage of labour. Is this true?

Some doctors describe a fourth stage of labour, referring to the time period after delivery of the placenta, while the uterus continues to contract. Uterine contraction is important in controlling bleeding after the birth of your baby.

The Three Stages of Labour

Stage	What's Happening	Your Experience	What you can Do
Stage 1 Early phase	• Uterine contractions cause cervix to dilate (open) and efface (thin out) • Cervix dilates to 1½–2in (4–5cm)	• Pinkish discharge ('show' or 'bloody show') • Membranes may rupture, causing a gush or trickle of amniotic fluid from your vagina • Mild contractions occur at 15–20 minute intervals in the beginning and last up to 1 minute. Gradually they become more regular and closer together	• To prevent vomiting, don't eat or drink anything once labour begins. • You may be able to stay at home for a while if you are at term. Ask your midwife or your doctor when you should to to the hospital. If it is preterm labour, if you have intense, constant pain or if you have bright red bleeding, call your doctor immediately. • Use relaxation and breathing techniques learned in childbirth class
Active phase	• Cervix dilates from1½in (4cm) to 3in (8cm) and continues to thin out	• Contractions are more intense and frequent • Contractions will be about 3 minutes apart and last about 45 seconds	• Continue using relaxation and breathing techniques • If labour is very painful, you may ask for an epidural
Transition phase	• Stage 1 is changing to Stage 2 • Cervix dilates from 3in (8cm) to 4in (10cm) and continues to thin out	• Contractions are 2–3 minutes apart and last about 1 minute and last about 1 minute • You may feel very strong pressure, causing the urge to push; don't push until your midwife or doctor says your cervix is completely dilated • You may be moved to delivery room	• Continue relaxation and breathing techniques to counteract urge to push

Stage	What's Happening	Your Experience	What you can Do
Stage 2	• Cervix is completely dilated • Baby continues to descend • As you push, your baby is born; the midwife or doctor will suction baby's nose and mouth, and clamp its umbilical cord	• Contractions occur at 2–5 minute intervals and last intervals and last 60–90 seconds • If you received an epidural, you may find it hard to push • You may have an episiotomy to prevent tearing of vaginal tissues as the baby is born	• After cervix is completely dilated, you will begin to push with each contraction • You may get gas and air (nitrous oxide and oxygen) to breathe.
Stage 3	• After the baby is born, the placenta separates from the wall of the uterus and is expelled • The midwife or doctor will examine placenta to ensure it is intact and all of it has been delivered • You may be given an injection of Syntometrine (oxytocin with ergometrine) or oxytocin to contract the uterus, help expel the placenta and reduce blood loss.	• Contractions may be closer together and less painful • Midwife or doctor will repair your episiotomy	• When baby is being delivered, listen to your midwife or doctor, who will tell you when and when not to push to prevent baby being born too quickly • As you push, you may able to watch your baby born if an overhead mirror is available • You'll meet and hold your baby • You may need to push to expel the placenta • You may be able to hold your baby while the midwife or doctor repairs your episiotomy

My sister-in-law said it's important for me to know how to contact my doctor or midwife when I go into labour. Why?

It's a good idea to ask your doctor certain questions about preparing to go into hospital. He or she may have specific instructions for you. You might want to ask your doctor or midwife the following questions.

• When should I go into hospital once I am in labour?
• Should I call you before I leave for the hospital?
• How can I reach you after regular surgery hours?
• Are there any particular instructions to follow during early labour?

My best friend told me she had a 'bloody show' just before she went into labour. What is it?

You may bleed a *small* amount of blood following a vaginal examination or at the beginning of labour. This bloody show occurs as the cervix stretches and dilates. If it causes you concern or appears to be a large amount of blood, contact your doctor or midwife immediately.

I read that I may pass a 'mucus plug' at the beginning of labour. Is this dangerous?

Along with a bloody show, you may pass some mucus, sometimes called a *mucus plug*. Passing this mucus doesn't always mean you'll have your baby soon or that your are beginning labour.

I've heard how important it is to time contractions once labour begins. Why?

There are two reasons for timing contractions:

• to find out *how long* a contraction lasts
• to find out *how often* contractions occur

It's important for your doctor or midwife to have this information so he or she can decide if it's time for you to go into hospital.

How do we time a contraction to find how long it lasts?

Begin timing when the contraction *starts*, and end timing when the contraction *lets up and goes away*.

How do we time a contraction to find how often it occurs?

Be sure to ask your doctor which method he or she prefers because there are two ways to time contractions.

- Start timing when the contraction *starts* and time it until the next contraction *starts*. This is the most common method.
- Start timing when the contraction *ends* and note how long it is until the next contraction *starts*.

What if I go into labour and my partner isn't with me?

Well before your delivery date, sit down and talk to your partner about how you will stay in touch as your due date approaches. Some of my patients rent personal pagers for the last few weeks for the partner to carry. Ask someone else to act as a back-up in case your partner cannot be with you or if you need someone to take you to the hospital.

I understand my partner can be very important during labour and delivery. How?

You partner can help in many ways. He can help prepare you for labour and delivery and can support you as you labour. He can share in the joy of the delivery of your baby. He can support you emotionally throughout the entire birthing process, which can be very important to you both.

What can a relative or friend do during labour and delivery?

A friend or relative who has had a baby can do a lot to help you through labour. She can:

- time your contractions so you are aware of the progress of your labour
- encourage and reassure you during labour
- help you deal with your physical discomfort
- help create a positive mood in the labour room
- report symptoms or pain to the doctor or midwife
- keep a watch on the door, and protect your privacy
- control traffic into your room

I've heard I can't drink anything during labour. Why?

Women often get nauseated, which may cause vomiting. It is for your safety that you are not allowed to eat or to drink anything during labour to keep your stomach empty.

If my labour is a long one, can I have anything to drink?

No, just sips of water or ice chips to suck on. If labour is long, you may be given fluids intravenously.

What about food – if my labour is extremely long, can't I eat something?
No, you can't. As I have explained, it's for your safety that you will not be allowed anything to eat.

I'm nervous about whether my baby is too big for me to deliver. Can my doctor tell before labour begins if I'll have problems?
Even with an estimation of how much your baby weighs, your doctor cannot really know if the baby is too big for you until after labour begins. Usually labour must begin so your doctor can see how the baby fits into your pelvis and if there is enough room for the baby to pass through the birth canal.

I've heard many different stories from friends, but I need an answer. Will I have to have an enema when I go into hospital to have my baby?
You may not be required to have an enema –it is usually a choice. You need to discuss this with your doctor or midwife at one of your antenatal appointments. There *are* benefits to having an enema early in labour. It decreases the amount of contamination by bowel movement or faeces during labour and at the time of delivery. It may also help you after delivery if you have an episiotomy because having a bowel movement very soon after delivery can be painful.

What can I expect when I have my first bowel movement after delivery?
Your first bowel movement usually occurs a day or two after delivery. If you had an enema, it could take a few days longer. It could be painful, especially if you have an episiotomy.

A friend said her doctor prescribed stool softeners for her, and they helped. Is this common?
Yes. Most doctors prescribe stool softeners after delivery to help with your bowel movements. They are safe to take, even if you are nursing.

What is occipito-posterior labour?
Occipito-posterior labour occurs when the baby comes out through the birth canal looking straight up. This type of presentation often causes lower-back pain.

If my baby is looking up, will that make my labour longer?
This type of labour may take longer for delivery. It may require rotation of the baby's head so it comes out looking down at the ground rather than up at the sky.

My sister-in-law had all sorts of friends present during her labour and when she gave birth last year. I don't want anyone but my husband with me. Is this unusual?
Whatever you want should be all right with your husband or partner. As I've said before, the birth experience can be stressful for you. As long as it's acceptable to your doctor, you should be allowed to make a lot of the decisions about the birth experience.

Tests during Labour

My doctor or midwife was mentioning fetal monitoring during labour and delivery. What is this?
In many hospitals, a baby's heart beat is monitored throughout labour, making it possible to detect any problems early so they can be resolved.

What kind of monitoring do they do?
There are two types of fetal monitoring during labour – *external fetal monitoring* and *internal fetal monitoring*.

What is external fetal monitoring?
This type of monitoring can be done before your membranes rupture. A belt with a receiver is strapped to your abdomen, and it records the baby's heartbeat. See the illustration opposite and the one on page 66.

What is internal fetal monitoring?
Internal fetal monitoring is a more precise method of monitoring the baby. An electrode is placed on the fetal scalp to record the fetal heart rate; it gives a more exact reading. See the illustration on page 67.

I recently read about fetal blood sampling during labour. What is this test?
It is another way of evaluating how well a baby is tolerating the stress of labour.

External contraction monitor

Monitor machine

External heart rate monitor

External monitoring during labour.

How is fetal blood sampling done during labour?

Membranes must be ruptured, and the cervix must be dilated at least ³/₄in (2cm). An instrument is applied to the scalp of the baby to make a small nick in the skin. The baby's blood is collected in a small tube, and its pH (acidity) is checked.

What can the doctor learn from fetal blood sampling?

The pH level can help determine whether the baby is having trouble during labour. Results help the doctor decide whether labour can continue or if a caesarean section needs to be done.

Dealing with the Pain of Childbirth

I've never had a baby before, and I'm terrified of the pain of childbirth. Is it really awful?

Childbirth *is* accompanied by pain; expectation of this pain can evoke fear and anxiety in you. This is normal. If you're concerned about pain and how you'll handle it, the best way to deal with it is to become informed about it.

My friend told me I won't feel like a 'real woman' unless I have my baby without any pain relief. Is this true?
Some women believe they'll feel guilty after their baby is born if they ask for pain relief during labour. Sometimes they believe the baby will be harmed by the medication. Some believe they'll deprive themselves of the complete birth experience. I tell my parents that the main goal of any labour and delivery is a *healthy baby*. If a woman needs pain relief to help her, it doesn't mean she's failed in any way!

How can I find out more about the different pain relief methods available during labour and delivery?
Discuss it with your doctor or midwife. Your childbirth preparation class is also a good place to ask about these drugs.

I've heard about 'analgesia' and 'anaesthesia' for pain relief. What's the difference?
Analgesia is pain relief without total loss of sensation. *Anaesthesia* is pain relief with total loss of sensation.

How does analgesia work?
An analgesic is injected into a muscle or vein to decrease the pain of labour, but it allows you to remain conscious. It provides pain relief but can make you drowsy, restless and nauseated. You may experience difficulty concentrating. it may slow the baby's reflexes and breathing, so it is usually given during the early and middle parts of labour.

How does anaesthesia work?
There are two types of anaesthesia – *general anaesthesia* and *local anaesthesia*, sometimes called *regional anaesthesia*. With general anaesthesia, you are completely unconscious, so it is used only for caesarean deliveries and emergency vaginal deliveries. Local anaesthesia affects a small area and is very useful for an episiotomy repair.

Is general anaesthesia dangerous?
There are some disadvantages to using a general anaesthesia – it is not used as much today as it was in the past. The advantage of general anaesthesia is that it can be administrated very quickly in an emergency. Disadvantages include causing the mother to vomit or to aspirate vomited food or stomach acid into her lungs.

Does local anaesthesia affect the baby?
Local anaesthesia rarely affects the baby and usually has few lingering effects.

I've heard there are several types of local anaesthesia. What are they?
The three most common types of local anaesthesia are pudendal block, spinal block and epidural block.

What is a pudendal block?
A *pudendal block* is having a drug injected into the vaginal area to relieve pain in the vagina, the perineum and the rectum. It allows the mother to remain conscious during its use. Side effects are rare. It is considered one of the safest forms of pain relief; however, it does not relieve uterine pain.

What is a spinal block?
With a *spinal block*, the drug is injected into spinal fluid in the lower back, which numbs the lower part of the body. The mother remains conscious during delivery with a spinal block. This type of block is administered only once during labour, so it is often used just before delivery. It works quickly and is an effective pain inhibitor.

What is an epidural block?
In an *epidural block*, a tube is inserted into a space outside the mother's spinal column in the lower back. A drug is administered through the tube for pain relief, and the mother remains conscious during delivery. The tube remains in place until after delivery so additional drugs can be administrated when necessary.

An epidural causes some loss of sensation in the lower part of the body. It helps relieve painful uterine contractions, pain in the vagina and rectum as the baby passes through the birth canal and the pain of an episiotomy. A woman can still feel pressure, so she can push adequately during vaginal delivery.

An epidural block is not effective in some women. Because an epidural may make it harder to push, vacuum extraction or forceps may be necessary during delivery.

What are the side effects of a spinal block or an epidural block?
Both a spinal block and an epidural block can cause a woman's blood pressure to drop suddenly, which in turn can cause a decrease in the

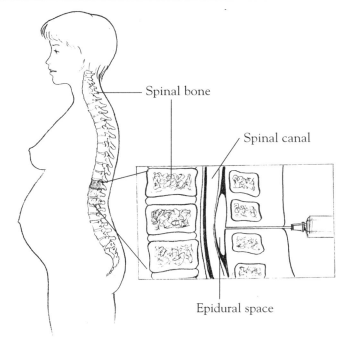

Epidural anaesthesia.

baby's heart rate. These blocks are not used if the woman is bleeding heavily or if the baby has an abnormal heart beat. A woman may experience a severe headache if the covering of the spinal cord is punctured during needle insertion with either type of anaesthesia.

I recently read about an anaesthesia called a 'walking spinal'. What is it?

A *walking spinal*, also called *intrathecal anaesthesia*, can be given to women who suffer extreme pain in the early stages of labour (less than 2in/5cm dilated). A small amount of narcotic, such as pethidine, is injected through a thin needle into the spinal fluid; this eases the pain and causes few side effects.

Because the dose is small, neither mother nor baby becomes overly drowsy. Sensory and motor functions remain intact, allowing the mother to walk around with help or sit in a chair.

Is a walking spinal available everywhere?

Unfortunately, its use at this time is very limited. Only a few teaching hospitals are using it. However, the number of places planning to use this type of anaesthesia may increase. Further testing is necessary before the procedure becomes routine and widely available.

Caesarean Section

My doctor has just told me I may need to have a caesarean section, and I'm scared. What is it exactly?
When a woman has a caesarean section, her baby is delivered through an incision made in the mother's wall and uterus.

Why is a caesarean section performed?
There are many reasons for doing a caesarean section, but the main goal of doing one is to deliver a healthy baby. Specific reasons include:

• a previous caesarean section
• to avoid rupture of the uterus
• the baby is too big to fit through the birth canal
• fetal distress
• compression of the umbilical cord
• baby is in the breech position
• placental abruption
• placenta praevia
• multiple fetuses – twins, triplets or more

I've read that more caesarean sections are being done today. Is this true?
There has been an increase in the rate of caesarean sections. In 1965, only 4 per cent of all deliveries were by caesarean section. Today between 10 and 20 per cent of all deliveries are caesarean sections.

Why are there more caesarean sections today?
We believe the increase is related to better monitoring during labour and safer procedures for caesarean sections. Women are also having bigger babies. A third factor in this increase may be rising malpractice rates and the fear of litigation. However, the goal is the same as it was before – a doctor wants to deliver the baby safely.

How is a caesarean section done?
An incision is made through the skin of the abdominal wall down to the uterus, and the wall of the uterus is cut. Then the amniotic sac

containing the baby and placenta is cut, and the baby is removed through the incisions. After the baby is delivered, the placenta is removed. The uterus is closed in layers with sutures that are absorbed (they don't have to be removed). The abdomen is then sewn together.

If I have to have a caesarean section, can I be awake?
With many caesarean sections, the anaesthetist will give you an epidural or a spinal anaesthetic. You are awake with these.

Can't my doctor tell if I'll need a caesarean section before I go into labour?
It would be nice to know this so you wouldn't have to go through labour, but it isn't that easy. We usually have to wait for labour contractions to see if your baby is stressed by them. And we have to wait to see if the baby will fit through the birth canal.

Are there any advantages to having a caesarean section?
The most important advantage is delivery of a healthy baby.

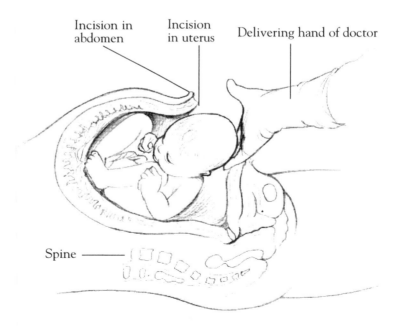

Incision in abdomen   Incision in uterus   Delivering hand of doctor

Spine

Caesarean section.

I'm sure there are disadvantages to having a caesarean section. What are they?
This is major surgery and carries with it certain risks, including infection, bleeding, shock through blood loss, the possibility of blood clots and injury to other organs, such as the bladder or rectum. You will probably have to stay in hospital a couple of extra days.

How long does it take to recover from caesarean section?
Recovery at home takes longer than it does with a vaginal delivery. The normal time for full recovery is 4 to 6 weeks.

How many caesarean sections can a woman have?
There is no exact number. Many doctors recommend no more than two or three, but this is evaluated at the time of each delivery. I have one patient on whom I recently performed her *eighth* caesarean section. This is unusual however.

Midline caesarean.

Bikini or pfannenstiel caesarean-section incision.

Some women at my childbirth preparation class said if you have a caesarean section, you've failed as a woman. Is this true?

No! If you have a caesarean section, you have *not* failed in any way! The goal in pregnancy, labour and delivery is a healthy baby and a healthy mother. In many situations, the *only* way to achieve that is with a caesarean section.

If a woman has repeat caesarean sections, how does the doctor perform the operation? Does he or she make a new, different incision for every birth?

Usually the same incision site will be used. If you have a large scar, your doctor may cut out the old scar.

I've heard that once you have a caesarean section, you must always have one. But don't some women deliver vaginally after having a caesarean section?

In the past it was felt that once a woman had a caesarean section, any later deliveries would have to be with the same operation. Today it is becoming quite common for women who have had a caesarean section to deliver vaginally with later pregnancies.

How does a woman know whether she can have a vaginal delivery after a caesarean section?

There are various factors that must be considered in making this decision. The type of incision done with the operation is important. With a classical incision, which goes high up on the uterus, labour is *not* permitted in subsequent pregnancies. If the woman is small and the baby is large, it may cause problems. Multiple fetuses and medical complications, such as diabetes or high blood pressure, may require a repeat caesarean section.

How many caesarean sections can I have and still be a candidate for vaginal delivery?

This is a matter for the judgement of your obstetrician. Most obstetricians will favour repeating a caesarean section after two previous caesarean sections. You should ask your obstetrician's advice and discuss his or her reasons with him or her.

What factors determine whether I can have a vaginal birth after having had a caesarean section?
Women who have the best chance of having a successful vaginal delivery after a caesarean section include women:

- whose original cause for a caesarean section is not repeated with the next pregnancy
- who have no major medical problems
- who had a low transverse incision (on the uterus) with their previous operation
- who have normal size babies
- whose babies are in the normal head-down position

If I want to try a vaginal delivery after a caesarean section, what can I do?
The most important thing to do is to discuss it with your doctor well in advance of labour so plans can be made. It may be helpful to get the records from your other delivery. Discuss the benefits and risks, and ask your doctor for his or her opinion as to your chances of a successful vaginal delivery. He or she knows your health and pregnancy history. Include your partner in this decision-making process.

Will I Need an Episiotomy?

What is an episiotomy?
An episiotomy is a surgical incision in the area behind the vagina, above the rectum; it is made during delivery to avoid tearing the vaginal opening or rectum.

Will my doctor require me to have an episiotomy?
This is something you need to discuss with your doctor at your antenatal visits. There are some situations that do not require an episiotomy, such as a small baby. Often this decision cannot be made until the time of delivery. An episiotomy may benefit a premature baby by avoiding pressure on the baby's head.

Does every woman have to have an episiotomy?
No, it is not necessary for everyone. Many women having their first or second baby will have an episiotomy. The more children a woman has had, the less likely it will be for her to need an episiotomy. It depends on the size of the baby.

My friend said she didn't need an episiotomy. Why does a woman have an episiotomy?
An episiotomy is done to allow room for the baby to fit through the birth canal and to avoid tearing other organs in the mother. Again, if a woman has had a few pregnancies and deliveries, she may not need a episiotomy with her later children.

What factors determine whether I have to have one?
Some factors leading to an episiotomy include:

• the size of the mother's vaginal opening
• the size of the baby's head and shoulders
• the number of babies previously delivered
• a forceps or vacuum delivery to avoid damage to the vulva, bladder and rectum

I've heard some episiotomies are bigger than others. What does this mean?
Description of an episiotomy includes a description of the depth of the incision. There are two degrees that describe incision depth:

• *1st degree* – cuts only the skin
• *2nd degree* – cuts the skin and underlying tissue, called fascia, and some of the muscles

How painful is an episiotomy?
After delivery of your baby, the most painful part of the entire birth process might be your episiotomy. Don't be afraid to ask for help with this pain. Many things can be done to help relieve it, including pain-relieving tablets or suppositories, ice, salt baths and laxatives.

The Baby's Birth Position

I heard a woman at the doctor's office say her baby was in a 'breech presentation'. What did she mean?
A *breech presentation* means the baby is not in a head-down position, and the legs or buttocks come into the birth canal first.

If my baby is in a breech presentation, is that bad?
Early in pregnancy, breech is common. By the last 4–6 weeks, your baby should be in a head-down position. If your baby is breech when it

is time to deliver, your doctor may try to turn the baby or you may need a caesarean section.

What causes a baby to be in a breech presentation?
One of the main causes is prematurity of the baby. Near the end of the second trimester, it's more common for the baby to present as a breech baby. As you progress through the third trimester, the baby usually turns into the head-down position for birth.

Are there different kinds of breech presentations and other abnormal positions?
Yes. There are three different breech presentations and two other abnormal positions:

* Frank breech – lower legs are flexed at the hips and extended at the knees. Feet are up by the face or head.
* Complete breech – one or both knees are flexed, not extended.
* Incomplete breech – a foot or knee enters the birth canal ahead of the rest of the baby.
* Face presentation – the baby's head is hyperextended so the face enters the birth canal first.
* Shoulder presentation – the baby is lying almost as if in a cradle in the pelvis. The head is on one side of the mother's abdomen and the bottom is on the other side.

How is a baby in the breech position delivered?
There is some controversy about this. For a long time, breech deliveries were performed vaginally, then it was believed the safest method was by caesarean section. Many doctors still believe a caesarean section is the safest way to deliver a baby in the breech position. However, some doctors believe a woman can deliver a breech baby without difficulty if the situation is right.

I've heard that sometimes the doctor will try to turn a baby in the breech position. Is that true?
Yes. If your baby is in a breech position, your doctor may attempt to change its position by using *external cephalic version*.

How is the baby turned?
The doctor places his or her hands on your abdomen. Using gentle movements, he or she manually shifts the baby into the head-down

position. An ultrasound scan is usually done first so the doctor can see the position of the baby. Ultrasound scanning is used during the procedure to guide the doctor in changing the baby's position.

When is external cephalic version usually done?
Most physicians who use this method do so before labour begins or in the early stages of labour.

How successful is external version?
It is successful in about 50 per cent of the cases in which it is used.

Can every doctor do external version?
Not every doctor is trained in the procedure, and some doctors do not believe it is of value.

Delivery of your Baby

How long does a vaginal delivery take?
The actual delivery of the baby and placenta (not including the labouring process) takes anywhere from a few minutes to an hour.

How long does a caesarean section take?
It usually takes from 30 to 60 minutes. However the part that takes the longest is not the birth of the baby – that is performed rather quickly. It is the stitching process to close the various skin and muscle layers after the baby is born that takes the greatest amount of time.

Will I deliver in the same room in which I labour?
That is the set-up in some hospitals. If you labour and deliver in the same room, then you may be able to remain there during recovery and for the rest of your stay at the hospital. Not all hospitals are equipped this way. In most, you will labour in a labour room and move to a delivery room to deliver. Then you will recover in a wardlike setting before being moved to your room, where you will remain until you go home.

I've read that there are other birth positions that are acceptable besides lying on my back. Is that true?
Yes there are. You may deliver lying on your side or squatting, if you make arrangements with your doctor or midwife to do this.

Will my doctor have to use forceps during the delivery?
It depends on the situation at the time of delivery. The factors involved include the size of the baby, the size of your pelvis, how well you are able to push and whether your baby needs to be delivered immediately.

Exactly what are forceps?
Forceps look like two metal hands which protect the baby's head and are used to help deliver the baby. However, they are not used as much today as the were in the past. Instead, doctors often use a vacuum extractor or perform a caesarean section.

What is a vacuum extractor?
A *vacuum extractor* is a plastic or metal cup that fits on the baby's head by suction. When you push during labour, your doctor is able to pull and help to deliver the baby more easily.

What is the Lamaze method of childbirth?
The *Lamaze method* provides education and practice for the mother and her partner in the weeks before birth. The woman learns breathing exercises to help her through her labour and learns ways to concentrate on objects to block out pain or to help reduce pain.

Can every woman use the Lamaze method?
The Lamaze method works very well for some women in labour. However, this approach requires a very serious commitment from the woman and her partner. It takes a great deal of practice and a lot of hard work during labour, but it can be very rewarding.

My partner wants to take a video of the birth, but I don't want him to. Am I being unreasonable?
No, you're not. The birth process is very private for many women, and they don't want to be videotaped, photographed or forced to share it with others. If this is your wish, explain it to your partner. He should respect your wishes. If he won't listen, discuss the problem with your doctor. Ask him or her to explain your objections to your partner.

After your Baby is Born

What happens to my baby after it is born?
First, the baby's mouth and throat are suctioned to clear out any secretions. Then the doctor clamps and cuts the umbilical cord. The baby is wrapped in clean blankets and may be placed on your abdomen. At 1 minute and 5 minutes after birth Apgar scores are recorded to show the baby's response to birth and to life on its own. An identity band is placed on the baby's wrist. Usually a brief physical examination or an assessment is done right after delivery. The baby may receive drops in its eyes to prevent infection and is given a vitamin K injection to prevent bleeding.

You may be asked if you want your baby to receive the hepatitis vaccine. You may have discussed this with your doctor. The vaccine is given to protect the baby against hepatitis in the future. However, you might decide not to have it given.

Once the initial evaluation is complete, the baby is returned to you. Later, the baby is placed in a heated bassinet for a period of time. See the chart on page 259 for a description of tests commonly performed on newborn babies.

My husband wants to cut the umbilical cord after the baby is delivered. Can he do this?
Talk to your doctor about your husband's participation in the delivery. What he is allowed to do varies from place to place.

I've heard my uterus will contract after my baby is born. How much will it shrink?
After you deliver your baby, the uterus shrinks from the size of a watermelon to the size of a volleyball. The uterus contracts and becomes smaller so it won't bleed.

How serious is bleeding after the birth of the baby?
You can expect to bleed after your delivery, but heavy bleeding is not very common. Bleeding is controlled by massaging the uterus and with injections of oxytocin or ergometrine; it lessens gradually over time then stops.

Is it normal to bleed heavily after my baby is born?
It's not unusual to lose a lot of blood during labour and delivery. However, heavy bleeding after the baby is born can be serious. A loss

of more than 18oz (500ml) in the first 24 hours after your baby's birth, called *postpartum haemorrhage*, is cause for concern.

What causes heavy bleeding?
The most common causes of heavy bleeding include the following:

• a uterus that won't contract
• tearing of the vagina or cervix during birth
• a large or bleeding episiotomy
• a tear, rupture or hole in the uterus
• failure of blood vessels inside the uterus to be compressed
• retained placental tissue
• clotting or coagulation problems

What is bleeding becomes heavy after a few days or weeks?
Contact your doctor. Sometimes the bleeding is normal, but it is best to talk to your doctor about it. He or she may want to see you to determine if the amount of bleeding is normal and, if necessary, to prescribe treatment.

I've heard that we can have the blood from our baby's umbilical cord saved and frozen for later use, if it is needed. Why would we want to do this?
Studies are being done on saving the blood in the umbilical cord for future use. Researchers are attempting to determine if the blood could be useful for various medical problems. For example, it might be helpful if your child develops leukaemia in the future. However, this is a very new practice and is not offered at very many hospitals at this time.

If your Baby is Late

What is a 'post dates birth'?
Babies born 2 weeks or more past their due date are called *post dates* or *post-term births*.

How common is post dates birth?
About 10 per cent of all babies are born more than 2 weeks past their due date.

Is a post dates birth dangerous for my baby?

The majority of babies born more than 2 weeks late are delivered safely. However, carrying a baby longer than 42 weeks can cause more problems for the fetus and the mother, so doctors conduct tests on these babies and induce labour, if necessary.

Why do they test a post dates baby?

A doctor can determine if a baby is moving around in the womb and if the amount of amniotic fluid is healthy and normal. If it is determined that the baby is healthy and active, the mother-to-be may be monitored until labour begins on its own. Tests are usually done as reassurance that an overdue baby is all right and can remain in the womb. These tests include a cardiotocogram (a fetal heart recording) and a biophysical profile. If signs of fetal stress are found, labour is often induced.

Emergency Childbirth

What should I do if I go into labour and can't make it to the hospital?

Emergency childbirth can happen to anyone, so the best thing to do is to be prepared. Read and study the information in the following boxes. Be sure you have the names and telephone numbers of your doctor or midwife and those of friends or family written down and near the phone. And if it happens to you, try to relax and follow the instructions provided.

Emergency Delivery at Home

1 Call 999 and ask for an ambulance.

2 Call a neighbour, family member or friend (have phone numbers available).

3 Encourage the woman *not* to push or to bear down.

4 Use blankets and towels to make the woman as comfortable as possible.

5 If there is time, wash the woman's vaginal and rectal areas with soap and water.

6 When the baby's head delivers, encourage the woman to pant or blow, and to concentrate on *not* pushing.

7 Try to ease the baby's head out with gentle pressure. Do not pull on the head.

8 After the head is delivered, gently push down on the head and push a little to deliver the shoulders.

9 As one shoulder delivers, lift the head up, delivering the other shoulder. The rest of the baby will quickly follow.

10 Wrap the baby in a clean blanket or towel.

11 Use a clean cloth or tissue to remove mucus from the baby's mouth.

12 Do not pull on the umbilical cord to deliver the placenta – it is not necessary.

13 If the placenta delivers on its own, wrap it in a towel or clean newspapers, and save it.

14 You don't need to cut the cord.

15 Keep the placenta at the level of the baby or above the baby.

16 Keep both mother and baby warm with towels or blankets until medical help arrives.

Emergency Delivery on the Way to the Hospital

1 Stop the car.

2 Try to get an ambulance. If you have a cellular phone dial 999.

3 Put on your flashing warning lights.

4 Place the woman in the back seat, with a towel or blanket under her.

5 Encourage the woman not to push or bear down.

6 When the baby's head delivers, encourage the woman to pant or blow, and to concentrate on *not* pushing.

7 Try to ease the baby's head out with gentle pressure. Do not pull on the head.

8 After the head is delivered, gently push down on the head and push a little to deliver the shoulders.

9 As one shoulder delivers, lift the head up, delivering the other shoulder. The rest of the baby will quickly follow.

10 Wrap the baby in a clean blanket or clean towels. Clean newspapers can be used if nothing else is available.

11 Use a clean cloth or tissue to remove mucus from the baby's mouth.

12 Do not pull on the umbilical cord to deliver the placenta – it is not necessary.

13 If the placenta delivers on its own, wrap it in a towel or clean newspapers and save it.

14 You don't need to cut the cord.

15 Keep the placenta at the level of the baby or above the baby.

16 Keep both mother and baby warm until you can get them to the hospital or medical help arrives.

Emergency Delivery if you are Alone

1 Call 999 and ask for an ambulance.

2 Call a neighbour, family member or friend (have phone numbers available).

3 Try not to push or bear down.

4 Find a comfortable place, and spread out towels or blankets.

5 If the baby comes before help arrives, try to use your hands to ease the baby out while you gently push.

6 Wrap the baby in a clean blanket or clean towels; hold it close to your body to keep it warm.

7 Use a clean cloth or tissue to remove mucus from the baby's mouth.

8 Do not pull on the umbilical cord to deliver the placenta – it is not necessary.

9 If the placenta delivers on its own, save it.

10 You don't need to cut the cord.

11 Try to keep yourself and your baby warm until medical help arrives.

PART IV

After your Baby is Born

CHAPTER 18

After your Baby's Birth

How long will I have to stay in hospital?
Most women are discharged within a day or two, if labour and delivery are normal and the baby is doing well. If you have a caesarean section, you need to stay a few days longer.

What can I expect during my recovery from a vaginal delivery?
Your blood pressure and bleeding will be checked closely for the first hours after the birth. You will be offered drugs for pain relief, and you will be encouraged to nurse your baby.

What can I expect during recovery if I have a caesarean section?
You will be in a recovery area where you will be monitored by a nurse. You will be offered medication for pain. After about an hour, you will be moved to your room.

I've heard the nurse will measure my urine output after delivery. Why?
This is checked to make sure your kidneys and bladder are working.

What is the pain after the childbirth like? What can I expect?
There are two main areas of pain – your abdomen and your episiotomy (if you have one). You can ask for pain relief tablets for both.

How can I tell if my episiotomy is all right?
It will be hard for you to tell. The midwives will check it for you.

What should I do if I get an infection in the episiotomy incision?
This type of infection is unusual and doesn't show up for a few days. It requires antibiotics for treatment.

If I don't want any more children, is it a good idea to have my tubes tied after I deliver my baby?
Some women choose to have a tubal ligation done while they are in hospital after the birth of their baby. However this is not the time to make a decision about tubal ligation if you haven't thought seriously about it before.

Are there advantages to having a tubal ligation after delivery?
Yes, there are. You are already in the hospital; if you have had an epidural, you already have the anaesthesia necessary for a tubal ligation.

What are the disadvantages to having a tubal ligation after delivering my baby?
Consider tubal ligation permanent and irreversible. If you have your tubes tied within a few hours or a day after having your baby, then change your mind, you will regret it. The failure rate, though very small is probably slightly higher than if the operation is done 3 months later.

If I didn't have an epidural, what kind of anaesthesia is used for a tubal ligation?
In most cases, it requires general anaesthesia.

Are there any activities I should avoid after my baby is born?
Avoid lifting any objects heavier than the baby for the first few weeks. If possible, avoid climbing stairs whenever you can.

I've decided not to breast feed. Will my doctor give me pills or an injection to dry up my milk?
You may be given pills to stop your milk from coming in, although it is not done as often now as was in the past. It is more common now to bind or wrap the breasts to stop the milk flow.

What if I decide I want to breast feed later. Can I?
No. If you stop your milk from coming in by taking medicine or not breast feeding, you won't be able to start it later.

My friend said she was really tired after her baby was born. Is this normal?
Many women are surprised by how tired they are, both emotionally and physically, in the first few months after the birth of the baby. Be sure to take time for yourself – you need a period of adjustment.

I've heard I should get lots of sleep after the baby is born. Why?
Sleep and rest *are* essential after the baby is born to help you get back in shape. To get the rest you need, go to bed early when possible. Try taking a nap or resting when the baby naps.

I feel exhausted having to deal with my baby. How can I get my husband to help me?
Parenthood is easier and more enjoyable when both partners share the responsibilities and chores. Couples should form an equal parenthood partnership. It will take a cooperative effort from both of you, but it can be done.

How do we form this partnership?
Try to sit down together *before* the baby is born and discuss what changes you are going to be facing. You may be able to avoid problems before they occur. Sharing tasks, such as bathing and nappy changing, seems to work out the best.

My mother told me that there are some warning signs of problems I may experience after birth. What are they?
You should not feel ill after birth. Call your doctor immediately if you have any of the following problems:

- unusually heavy or sudden increase in vaginal bleeding (more than your normal menstrual flow or soaking more than two sanitary pads in 30 minutes)
- vaginal discharge with strong, unpleasant odour
- a temperature of 100.6°F (38°C) or more, except for the first 24 hours after birth
- breasts that are painful or red
- loss of appetite for an extended period of time
- pain, tenderness, redness or swelling in your legs
- pain in the lower abdomen or in the back

What are 'after-baby blues'?

The term *after-baby blues* refers to a feeling of depression a woman may experience after her baby is born. It is also called *postpartum depression*. The condition is marked by anxiety, crying, depression, irritability and restlessness. It is often worst on the 4th day after delivery. It sometimes lasts a week or two and is caused by the change in hormone levels in a woman's body after her baby is born.

What can I do about after-baby blues?

If you don't feel better in a few days, call your doctor. Discuss your concerns with him or her; you'll be advised what to do. You may be referred to outside help, if it is needed. If you don't take care of yourself, your depression can worsen and can affect your physical health as well as your relationships with your baby and your partner.

Will I ever regain the tightness of my abdominal skin now that my baby is born?

For some women, skin returns to normal naturally. For others, it never returns to its prepregnancy state. Abdominal skin is not like muscle, so it can't be strengthened by exercise. One of the main factors that affects your skin's ability to return to its prepregnancy tightness is connective tissue, which provides suppleness and elasticity. As you get older, your skin loses connective tissue and elasticity. Other factors include your state of fitness before pregnancy, heredity and how greatly your skin was stretched during pregnancy.

My breasts grew quite a bit during pregnancy. Will they return to their normal size?

Most women find their breasts return to their prepregnancy size or decrease a little in size. This is a result of the change in the connective tissue that forms the support system in a woman's breasts. Exercise will not make breasts firmer, but it can improve the chest area so breasts have better support.

I thought I'd feel thinner now that I'm no longer pregnant, but I still feel fat. What can I do about my weight?

It's normal to lose 10–15lb (4.5–6.75kg) immediately after your baby is born. Extra weight may be harder to lose. Your body stored about 7–10lb (3.15–4.5kg) of fat to provide energy for the first few months after birth. If you eat properly and get enough exercise, these pounds will slowly come off.

Shouldn't I go on a strict diet to lose the weight?
No! Don't go on a strict diet right away – wait until later. Even if you don't breast feed your baby, your body requires a well-balanced, nutritious diet for you to stay healthy and keep your energy levels up.

I've heard I shouldn't diet if I'm breast feeding. Why?
All the nutrients your baby receives while breast feeding depends on the quality of the food you eat. Breast feeding places more demands on your body than pregnancy. Your body burns up to 1,000 calories a day just to produce milk. When breast feeding, you need to eat an extra 500 calories a day. Be sure to keep fluid levels up.

I really want to get back to exercising now that my baby is born. How should I approach exercising?
Exercise is important to your total feeling of well-being. Do something you enjoy, and do it on a regular basis. Walking and swimming are excellent exercises to help you get back in shape. However, before you start any postnatal exercise programme, be sure to check with your doctor. He or she may have some particular advice for you.

I want to get in shape as soon as possible, now that my baby's born. What can I do?
Be careful about beginning an exercise programme too soon. Discuss it with your doctor first. Be sure you don't overtire yourself. Get adequate rest.

What kind of activities can I start with?
Walking is a good exercise, but take it slowly. Ask your doctor when and how you can increase your exercise programme.

Your Postnatal Check up

I'm scheduled for a postnatal check up in 6 weeks. Do I really need to go?
Yes. Your postnatal check up is the last part of a complete pregnancy care programme. It is just as important as seeing your doctor or midwife during pregnancy. A postnatal check up is scheduled between 2 and 6 weeks after delivery, depending on the circumstances of the birth.

What will my postnatal check up cover?

You will have a physical examination, similar to the one at your first antenatal examination. Your doctor will also do an internal examination. If you had any birth tears or incisions, your doctor will examine them to see how they are healing. This is a good time to discuss birth control, if you haven't already made plans.

Why do I have to have a pelvic examination now that my baby is born?

Your doctor does an internal examination to determine if your uterus is returning to its prepregnant size and position. This normally takes about 6 weeks. If there are any problems, they can be taken care of at this time.

Birth Control after Pregnancy

When can I resume sexual relations with my partner?

Four to six weeks after delivery, if your recovery is normal.

I've heard that breast feeding is a good way to keep from getting pregnant. Is this true?

Breast feeding decreases your chances of getting pregnant, but you *cannot* rely on breast feeding or the lack of menstruation to protect you against getting pregnant again. You need to use some type of protection when you resume intercourse.

What type of birth control can I use while breast feeding?

There are many types of contraception you can use – condoms, birth-control foam or jelly, diaphragms, coils, Norplant. Talk about your options with your doctor.

Should I talk to my doctor about contraception at my postnatal check up?

This is the perfect time to discuss it. If you are not planning another pregnancy immediately, you need to discuss this with your doctor. You can ask about contraceptive methods. You may decide on oral contraceptives, Norplant or a coil. You will need a prescription for an oral contraceptive. If you decide on Norplant or a coil, you will have to make arrangements for the procedure.

I've heard I can't use birth control pills while I'm breast feeding. Why?
The amounts of hormones in routine oral contraceptives that pass into
breast milk are very small indeed, but some doctors think breast milk
production is reduced. Most doctors think a 'progestogen-only' pill
(Micronor) is without any ill effects used postnatally. Otherwise
choose some other form of contraception while breast feeding, such as
condoms or a diaphragm.

Making your Home Safe for the Baby

***I recently heard on television that baby-proofing a house is
important, even when the baby is very young. What did they mean?***
First, you cannot baby-proof a house. All you can do is make it baby-
safe. Accidents can and do happen, so it's best to try to safeguard your
baby's environment. Keep in mind the following.

- Cot slats should be no further apart than 2³/₈in (6cm).
- Be sure the mattress fits securely.
- Keep the cot away from windows, wall decorations, heating units,
  climbable furniture, blind and curtain cords, and other possible dangers.
- Never use a pillow in the cot.
- Keep the side up and locked when the baby is in the cot.
- Keep mobiles and other cot toys out of the baby's reach. You may
  have to remove them as the baby grows older.
- Never hang a pacifier or anything else around your baby's neck.
- Never leave the baby unattended on a sofa, chair, changing table or
  any other surface above the floor.
- Never put a baby seat on a work surface or table.
- Use safety straps with all baby equipment.
- Never leave a baby unattended in *any* water. A baby can drown in
  1in (2.5cm) of water.
- Never hold your baby while you're cooking or drinking any hot
  beverage.
- If you warm formula or baby food in the microwave, it can heat
  unevenly, causing hot spots. Be sure to shake the bottle or stir the
  food well before serving.
- Don't hang anything on stroller handles, such as a purse or bag. The
  extra weight could cause the stroller to tip over.
- Always put your baby in a car seat, even for a very short ride. Be sure
  the car seat is safety approved and installed correctly.

CHAPTER 19

Your New Baby

I've heard that my baby will have to have a lot of tests after it's born. What are they?
After delivery, the hospital staff conduct a variety of tests to evaluate your baby. The choice of test depends on your medical history, findings obtained during examination of the newborn and other factors. Tests performed on the baby include:

- Apgar test
- screening for hyperphenylketonuria, anaemia and hypothyroidism
- Coombs' test
- reflex assessment
- assessment of neonatal maturity
- other blood tests

See the chart opposite for an explanation of these tests.

Someone said there are differences in the birth weight of babies. Can you tell me more about it?
Yes, we've found three distinct differences in the birth weight of babies. However, these are general statements and do not apply in all cases.

- Boys weigh more than girls.
- Birth weight of a baby increases with the increasing number of pregnancies or babies you deliver.
- White babies at term weigh more than black babies at term.

Tests on the Newborn

Test	How Test is Performed	What Test Indicates
Apgar test	At 1 and 5 minutes after birth, baby is assessed for colour, heart rate, muscle tone, reflex response, breathing. Each category receives a score from 0 to 2 points, for a maximum of 10 points.	Gives an indication of baby's general condition at birth. Helps hospital staff decide if newborn needs extra care. Does not indicate what the future may hold.
Blood tests	Blood is taken from baby's heel.	Detects phenylketonuria, anaemia and hypothyroidism.
Coombs' test	Blood is taken from umbilical cord if mother's blood is rhesus negative, type O or has not been tested for antibodies.	Detects whether rhesus antibodies have been found.
Reflex assessment	Tests several specific reflexes, including the rooting and grasp reflexes.	If a particular reflex is not present, further evaluation is necessary.
Assessment of neonatal maturity	Many characteristics of baby are assessed to evaluate neuromuscular and physical maturity.	Each characteristic is assigned a score; sum indicates infant's maturity.
Other blood tests	Blood is taken from heel to test for sickle-cell anaemia, blood glucose levels or other problems.	Results indicate whether baby needs further evaluation.

Your Newborn's Appearance

What does the baby look like at birth?
The baby is wet and usually has some blood on it. Vernix, a white or yellow waxy substance, may cover part or much of its body.

I always thought all newborn were beautiful, but my new baby isn't very pretty. Her head looks too big. What's wrong with her?
A baby's head is large in proportion to the rest of her body. At birth, it measures one-quarter of her entire length. As she grows, this will change until her head is one-eighth of her adult height.

My little girl looks as if she's been in a fight – her nose is flat and lumpy. Will she need plastic surgery?
The shape of your little girl's nose at birth has little to do with what it will look like when she's an adult. A newborn's nose may look too flat to breathe through, but babies manage to breathe through them.

My little boy's head is misshapen. Will it always be like this?
If your baby made his appearance into this world through the birth canal, he may have an elongated head. The shape is only temporary and will become more 'normal' in the next few days.

My husband and I each have lots of hair, but our son is completely bald. Our daughter had lots of hair when she was born. Why the difference?
Your baby may be born with lots of hair or none at all. Don't worry about it. If he has lots of hair, this first hair will fall out during the first 6 months and will be replaced by hair that may be entirely different in colour and texture. If he doesn't have any hair, it's not a permanent condition either. He will eventually grow hair.

My baby's eyes seem to be swollen. What causes this?
A newborn's eyes are often swollen or puffy immediately after birth. This is caused by pressure in the birth canal and subsides in a few days.

When they brought my baby to me in my room, his eyes looked greasy and were kind of red. What did they do to him?
Your baby's eyes may have been slightly irritated and reddened by drops or ointment applied to his eyes shortly after birth. This is sometimes used to prevent eye infections. Redness usually disappears within 48 hours after birth.

My little girl has one eye that seems to wander when she looks at me. Is this an indication of some major problem?

One of your baby's eyes may wander when she looks at you, or she may look cross-eyed. Don't worry. Her eye muscles aren't strong enough yet to control her eye movements. A wandering eye usually corrects itself by the time the baby is 6 months old. If she still has a problem after that, discuss it with your doctor.

My little boy looks as if he's squinting at me. Are his eyes all right?

The skin folds at the inner corners of his eyes make it look as if he's squinting. As time passes, these folds become less prominent, and he won't look as if he's squinting any more.

My baby's skin seems dry and flaky. I had always heard a baby's skin was soft and beautiful. Should I be concerned?

Within hours after birth, a baby's skin begins to dry out and may become flaky and scaly. This can last for a few weeks after birth. You really don't need to treat it, but you may want to rub a little lotion on your baby's delicate skin.

A friend told me my baby will probably get a lot of different rashes. Is this normal?

It is normal for babies to get various types of rash in the first few months after birth. Don't be too alarmed about them. Contact your doctor if any rash lasts longer than a few days or if your baby seems to be extremely uncomfortable.

What kinds of rashes can I expect my baby to get?

A baby may develop the following rashes.

- *Nappy rash.* This is the most common type. Keep the area dry and clean, and apply a protective ointment that contains zinc oxide.
- A red, blistery rash may be *prickly heat.* Apply cornstarch to the affected area, and don't overdress the baby.
- Tiny yellow bumps on the face, called *milia*, affect about half of all newborns.
- Large yellow pimples on splotchy skin is called *newborn rash.* This affects about 70 per cent of all newborns.
- Swollen pink pimples are called *newborn acne.*

Treatment for milia, newborn rash and newborn acne is time – you don't need to do anything. They will disappear on their own in a short time.

I know a baby's skin is sensitive. Is it all right to take my baby out in the sun?

It's best to avoid exposing your baby to sunlight. A newborn's skin has little or no ability to protect itself from damage by the sun. Sunscreens are not recommended for babies under 6 months, so keep your little one in the shade for the best protection. Put a hat and protective clothing on the baby for even a brief outing in the sun, especially in very hot, sunny areas.

Your Baby's Health

I've never had a baby before. I'm concerned that I won't know when he's ill or when I should call the doctor. Do you have any recommendations?

If your baby exhibits any of the following symptoms, call your doctor:

- fever higher than 100.6°F (38°C)
- inconsolable crying for long periods of time
- problems with urination
- projectile vomiting, in which stomach contents come out with great force
- baby appears lethargic or floppy when held
- severe diarrhoea
- unusual behaviour
- poor appetite

Any of these could be an indication that your baby is ill.

My brother's baby suffers from ear infections. I'm uncertain I'll be able to tell if my baby has an ear infection. What should I look for?

It may be difficult for you to determine that your baby has an ear infection. Symptoms that my indicate an ear infection in babies under 6 months of age include:

- irritability that lasts all day
- sleeplessness
- lethargy
- feeding difficulties

These symptoms may be hard to discern and may not be accompanied by fever. For babies between 6 and 12 months of age, symptoms are similar, except that fever is more common. The onset of ear pain may be sudden, acute and more noticeable.

I understand that dehydration is extremely dangerous in a baby. How will I know if my baby is dehydrated?
Dehydration in an infant can be *very* serious. If it occurs, call your doctor immediately. There are some warning signs to watch for.

• Baby wets fewer than six cloth or five disposable nappies a day.
• Baby's urine is dark yellow or orange. It should be pale yellow.
• Baby has fewer than two loose stools a day.
• Baby seems to be having trouble sucking.
• The soft spot on baby's head is sunken in.
• Baby is listless or otherwise unhealthy.

I've heard it's dangerous for a baby to have diarrhoea. How will I know if my baby has diarrhoea?
If you are concerned, call your doctor. A change in the number of nappies used or the consistency of the bowel movement is the first clue.

What should I do if my baby has diarrhoea?
The first thing to do is call your doctor. If your baby has diarrhoea, he or she will need extra water and minerals to prevent dehydration. Your doctor may recommend an oral electrolyte solution to help replenish your baby's lost fluids and minerals.

Jaundice

I've heard about newborns with jaundice. What is jaundice?
Jaundice is the yellow staining of the skin, sclera (eyes) and deeper tissues of the body. It is caused by the newborn's inability to handle *bilirubin*, a chemical produced in the liver.

Is jaundice dangerous for a newborn?
Yes. Jaundice is caused by too much bilirubin in the baby's blood, a condition called *hyperbilirubinaemia*. It can be dangerous for the baby if it is left untreated. Problems for the baby may include central nervous system damage (brain damage) or *kernicterus* (very high hyperbilirubinaemia). Kernicterus can result in spasticity, lack of coordination in muscles, mental retardation and even death.

How is jaundice diagnosed?

The baby's colour is observed by the paediatrician and the nurses in the baby nursery. The baby looks yellow because of the excess amounts of bilirubin in the blood.

How is it treated?

Phototherapy is the treatment of choice for jaundice. The baby is placed under special lights; the light penetrates the baby's skin and destroys the bilirubin. In more severe cases, exchange blood transfusions may be necessary.

Colic

Both of my sister's babies had colic. What is it exactly?

Colic is a condition marked by episodes of loud, sudden crying and fussiness, which can often last for hours, in a baby that is otherwise healthy. About 20 per cent of all babies experience the pain and crying caused by colic. In full-blown colic, the abdomen becomes distended and the infant passes wind often.

What should I do if I think my baby may have colic?

The only way to know if your baby has colic is to see your family doctor. He or she can determine if it is colic or if your baby is having some other problem.

When does colic appear?

It usually appears gradually in the baby about 2 weeks after birth. As days pass, the condition worsens, then often disappears around the age of 3 months but occasionally lasts until 4 months. Colic attacks usually occur at night beginning in the late afternoon and early evening and last 3 to 4 hours. The attacks cease as quickly as they begin.

What causes colic?

Researchers have been studying colic and its causes for a long time, but we still have little proof why it occurs. Theories about its causes include:

- immaturity of the digestive system
- intolerance to cow's milk protein in formula or breast milk
- fatigue in the baby

If our baby suffers from colic, what can we do?

At this time, we cannot offer a definitive answer on ways to stop the colic. Most doctors recommend using a variety of methods to try to ease the baby's discomfort.

- Offer the baby the breast or a bottle of formula.
- Try 'non-cow's' milk formula, if you bottle feed.
- Carry your baby in a sling during an attack. Motion and closeness often help somewhat.
- Put the baby on its stomach across your knees and rub its back.
- Wrap the baby snugly in a blanket.
- Massage or stroke the baby's tummy.

Your Baby's Sleeping Habits

I've heard stories about how difficult it is to get a baby to go to sleep at night. What can I do about this?

The wisest thing is to establish a routine to help your baby develop healthy sleeping habits.

- Wait until your baby is tired before you put him to bed.
- Develop a regular, predictable routine for bed.
- Develop good sleep associations, such as a favourite blanket or toy. Don't put your baby to bed with a bottle!
- Never leave your baby alone on a water bed.

My brother's new baby wants to sleep all day and stay up all night. Is there any way to get a baby to sleep at night and be up during the day?

There are some things a parent can do to try to change the day/night situation with the baby.

- Limit daytime naps to a few hours each.
- Don't overstimulate the baby when you get up for night feedings.
- By day, let your baby nap in a light area, with some noise. At night, put him or her in a very quiet, dark room to sleep.
- Keep your baby up during the day by talking and singing or providing other stimulation.

I heard that it's better to put a baby down to sleep on its side or back, rather than on its stomach. Is this true?
Research has proved that it *is* better to place a baby on its side or back when putting it down to sleep. We have discovered this position greatly reduces the incidence of SIDS (sudden infant death syndrome or 'cot death').

Someone told me that there's a difference in the sleep habits between bottle fed and breast fed babies. Is this true?
Yes, it is. Sleep patterns develop differently for bottle fed and breast fed babies. Bottle fed babies sleep longer at night as they mature. Breast fed babies don't shift to longer sleep patterns until around the time they are weaned. See the chart below for a comparison of bottle fed and breast fed babies' sleep patterns.

Taking Care of your Baby

I'm nervous about dealing with the baby's umbilical cord. What should I do?
It isn't that difficult to deal with the stump of the umbilical cord. It will fall off 7 to 10 days after birth. Until it does, clean your baby with sponge baths instead of tub baths.

My baby's eyes are all gooey. How can I safely clean them?
To remove 'sleep' from your baby's eyes, use a moistened cotton ball. Place the cotton ball at the inner corner of the eye, and wipe vertically down the nose.

Length of Night-time Sleep Patterns

	Bottle fed Babies	*Breast fed Babies*
Newborn	5 hours	4 to 7 hours
4 months	8 to 10 hours	4 to 7 hours
6 months	9 to 10 hours	4 to 7 hours
Total sleep in 24 hours	13 to 15 hours	11 to 14 hours

How can I clean my baby's nose?
Never put anything inside your baby's nose. If you need to remove dried nasal secretions, gently wipe around the nose. Dried nasal secretions are usually sneezed out.

Is there an easy way to clean my baby's ears?
Never probe in your baby's ears with any object! Ear wax is there for a purpose. It's all right to clean around the outside of the ears with a soft washcloth, but don't put anything inside your baby's ears.

I've been trying to decide between cloth and paper nappies for my new baby. Is one better than the other?
This is a tough question to answer because you must take into consideration your lifestyle, budget and baby. *Disposable nappies* are very convenient. You don't need pins or plastic pants, and you never have to wash them. *Cloth nappies* can be used many times. Some styles don't need pins or plastic pants. You will need adequate washing and drying facilities, or you may choose a nappy service. Many of my patients use a combination of disposable and cloth nappies.

My little girl was big when she was born, and I don't want her to be fat. Should I be concerned about how fat she is now?
No, that's not really a concern at this early age. You should focus on whether your baby is growing and developing appropriately, not how fat she is. Do *not* put your baby on a diet to keep her slim!

Will my doctor tell me if my baby is too fat?
Your doctor will be more concerned about where your child fits on the growth charts in relation to other children. Usually a child's weight (and height) are given using a percentile. For example, if you are told your daughter is in the 80th percentile, it means 80 out of 100 children weigh less than she does and 20 children weigh more.

Is there any way I can keep my baby from being obese?
There are some tips to help you give your baby the best nutritional start possible.

• Breast feed your baby.
• Do not introduce solid foods until the age of 4 to 6 months.
• Feed your baby in response to hunger, not to meet other needs or just because it's 'time to eat'.

• Encourage physical activity and sound eating habits for everyone in your family.

Car Restraints – For the Safety of your Baby

Does my baby need to ride in a car safety-restraint seat all the time?
Every time your baby rides in the car, he or she should be in an approved safety-restraint seat. In an accident, an unrestrained child becomes a missile-like object. The force of a crash can literally pull a child out of an adult's arms!

What about short trips, like going home from the hospital – what can happen to my baby?
It's incredible, but one study showed more than 30 deaths a year occur to unrestrained babies *going home from the hospital after birth!* In nearly all these cases, if the baby had been in an approved infant-restraint system, he or she would have survived the accident. Don't take chances – keep your baby safely restrained.

My mother said that it's against the law to let babies ride in a car without a safety-restraint system. Is this true?
No, it isn't. Parents are not legally obliged to fit a baby's car seat in their car. However, it is strongly recommended that they do and that the baby is safely restrained on every journey, no matter how short.

Where is the safest spot in the car to put the baby's car seat?
The safest spot is in the middle of the back seat. In this position, it is more protected in the event of a side collision. Manufacturers recommend *not* putting the car seat in the front of the car if you have a passenger-side air bag. If the bag inflates, it can knock the car seat around or even injure the baby.

CHAPTER 20

Feeding your Baby

How will I know when my baby is hungry?
A baby exhibits definite signs of hunger, including:

- fussing
- putting the hands in the mouth
- turning the head and opening the mouth when a cheek is touched

How often does a baby need to feed?
Early in life, most babies need to feed every 3 to 4 hours, although some babies feed as often as every 2 hours. It may help your baby to get on a schedule if you feed at regular intervals. Or you can let your baby set your schedule – some babies need to nurse more often than others. Sometimes your baby will need to feed more often than he or she usually does. See how often your baby wants to feed and whether he or she is growing properly. These are the best guides to feeding your baby. Usually, as time goes by, the baby waits longer between feedings and feeds longer at each feeding.

How much should I feed my baby at each feeding?
A baby is usually the best judge of how much he or she should take at each feeding. Usually a baby will turn away from the nipple (mother or bottle) when it is full.

I've heard that babies don't need to be fed breast milk or formula every time they're thirsty, that water is all right sometimes. How do I know when I should give water?
Discuss this with your doctor or midwife. Much depends on your baby's weight, how well he or she is doing and whether he or she is hungry or

thirsty. Your doctor will give you answers.

Do all babies need to be burped?
It's a good idea to burp your baby after each feeding. Some babies need to be burped during a feeding as well. Hold your baby over your shoulder or sit your baby in your lap, and gently rub or pat the back. You will probably want to place a towel over your shoulder or at least have one handy in case he or she spits up. If your baby doesn't burp, don't force it.

Is spitting up common in babies?
It is common during the early months of life because the muscle at the top of the stomach is not yet fully developed. When a baby spits up enough to propel the stomach contents several inches, it is called *vomiting*. If your baby vomits after a feeding, do not feed him or her again immediately – the stomach may be upset. It may be wise to wait until the next feeding.

Is it true breast feeding is the best choice for my baby?
If you can breast feed, we have found it is best for the baby. Breast milk contains all the nutrients a baby needs, and it's easy to digest. Breast fed babies have lower rates of infections because of the antibodies in breast milk. And breast feeding provides the baby with a sense of security and the mother with a sense of self-esteem. However, if there are reasons you cannot or choose not to breast feed, be assured that your baby will do well on formula.

My sister had problems and couldn't breast feed. What if something like that happens to me and I can't breast feed – will it harm my baby?
No, it will not harm your baby if you cannot or choose not to breast feed. I don't want any mother to feel guilty because she doesn't breast feed her baby. Sometimes you cannot breast feed because of some physical condition or other problem. Sometimes you choose not to breast feed because of other demands on your time, such as a job or other children to care for. Your baby can still get all the love and attention *and* nutrition it needs if breast feeding is not possible for you.

Bottle Feeding as One Option

I may be in the minority, but I want to bottle feed, not breast feed. Will I be a terrible mother because I feel this way?
No, you will not be a terrible mother because you choose not to breast feed. In fact, statistics show that more women choose to bottle feed than breast feed their babies. We know that, through the use of iron-fortified formula, your baby can receive good nutrition if you bottle feed. So don't berate yourself or feel guilt if you bottle feed – it's a personal decision that *you* must make.

I've heard all the great things about breast feeding. Aren't there any good things to be said about bottle feeding?
There *are* advantages to bottle feeding that are often overlooked. Some women enjoy the freedom that bottle feeding provides. Someone else can help care for the baby. Fathers can be more involved in the care of the baby. Bottle fed babies are often able to last longer between feedings because formula is usually digested more slowly than breast milk. And you can determine exactly how much formula your baby is taking in at each feeding.

I've definitely decided I want to bottle feed. Is there any special way to bottle feed a baby?
Try to build these steps into your bottle feeding routine.

- Snuggle your baby close to you during feeding.
- Heat the formula to body temperature by running under warm water.
- Place the bottle's nipple right side up, ready to feed.
- Don't touch the tip of the nipple.
- Brush the nipple lightly over the baby's lips, and guide it into the baby's mouth. Don't force it.
- Tilt the bottle so the neck is always filled, keeping the baby from sucking in too much air.
- Remove the bottle during feeding to let the baby rest. It usually takes 10 to 15 minutes to finish feeding.
- Don't leave the baby alone with the bottle. *Never* prop up a bottle and leave the baby alone to suck on it.
- Never put a baby down to bed with a bottle.

Do I have to warm up the formula before I feed it to my baby?
There's no evidence that feeding refrigerated formula without warming it will harm your baby. If you usually warm it, your baby will probably prefer it that way. If your baby is usually breast fed, he or she will probably prefer a warmed bottle. Be careful formula is not *too hot.*

I'm concerned about which formula to use. Are there different types?
Yes, there are. Most babies do very well on milk-based formula, but some babies need specialised formulas.

What types of formula are there besides the normal milk-based ones?
Several types are available on the market today, including:

. *milk-based, lactose-free formula* – fed to babies with feeding problems caused by lactose intolerance, such as fussiness, wind and diarrhoea.
. *soya-based formula* – milk-free and lactose-free for babies with milk allergies or sensitivity
. *hypoallergenic protein formula* – easier to digest and lactose-free for babies with colic or other symptoms of milk-protein allergy

I recently read that it is better for the baby to bottle feed with a bottle that is slanted. Why?
Research has shown that feeding a baby with a bottle that is slanted is better. This design keeps the nipple full of milk, which means baby takes in less air. A slanted bottle also helps ensure baby is sitting up to drink. When a baby drinks lying down, milk can pool in the eustachian tube, where it can cause ear infections.

How long should a baby receive formula?
Some paediatricians recommend that a baby be fed iron-fortified formula for the first year of life. Feeding for this length of time helps maintain adequate iron intake.

Breast feeding as your other Option

When can I begin breast feeding?
You can usually begin breast feeding your baby within an hour after birth. This provides your baby with *colostrum*, the first milk your breasts produce. Colostrum contains important factors that help boost the baby's resistance to infection. Breast feeding also causes your

pituitary gland to release oxytocin, a hormone that causes the uterus to begin contracting and to stop bleeding.

I'm nervous about breast feeding. How do I start?
Don't be discouraged if you don't feel natural at first. It takes some time to find out what will work best for you and your baby. Hold the baby across your chest, or lie in bed, making sure that he or she can reach the breast easily. Your baby should take your nipple into the mouth fully, so that the baby's gums cover the areola. He or she can't suck effectively if your nipple is only partly drawn into the mouth.

I've heard that breast feeding is the best way to bond with my baby. Is this true?
Breast feeding is an excellent way to bond with your baby because of the closeness between mother and child established during the feeding process. However, there are also other ways you can bond with your baby. Studies have shown that carrying your baby close to your body in a sling-like carrier helps the bonding process. It's great because dads can bond this way with baby, too.

I read that breast feeding can prevent milk allergies. How?
It's nearly impossible for a baby to become allergic to its mother's breast milk. This is important if there is a history of allergies in your family or your partner's family. The longer a baby breast feeds, the less likely he or she is to be exposed to substances that could cause allergic problems.

Everyone always mentions the good things about breast feeding. What are some of the disadvantages?
The greatest disadvantage for many mothers is the fact they are tied down to the baby so completely. They must be available when their baby is hungry. Breast feeding can also make other family members feel left out. Mothers who breast feed must pay careful attention to their diet, both for the nourishment they take in and the avoidance of foods that pass into their breast milk and cause problems for the baby. Also, caffeine, alcohol and some medicines can pass into breast milk.

I've heard stories about friends having to be up half the night to breast feed? How long does it usually take for a baby to nurse?
Usually most babies will breast feed every 2 to 3 hours for 5 to 15 minutes per breast.

How Breast Feeding Affects You

Someone told me I had to drink lots of fluids (water mostly) while I'm breast feeding. Is this true?
It's a good idea to keep up your fluid intake if you breast feed.

Can I diet if I'm breast feeding?
No, it's best not to diet while breast feeding. All the nutrients your baby receives from breast feeding depend on the quality of the food *you* eat. Breast feeding places more demands on your body than pregnancy. Your body burns up to 1,000 calories a day just to produce milk. When breast feeding, you need to eat an extra 500 calories a day, and be sure to keep fluid levels up.

I've heard that breast feeding is a good way to keep from getting pregnant? Is this true?
No. Do *not* rely on breast feeding to protect you against getting pregnant again. You need to use some type of protection when you resume intercourse.

My doctor said I shouldn't use birth control pills while I'm breast feeding. Why?
Do not use routine oral contraceptives if you are breast feeding. Some doctors think they reduce breast milk production. Tiny amounts of the hormones in oral contraceptives can get into your milk and be passed along to your baby, though it is doubtful if they can affect the baby's development. Progestogen-only oral contraceptives (Micronor) are prescribed by many doctors for breast feeding mothers but you may wish to use some other form of birth control until you have finished breast feeding.

My sister told me not to eat spicy foods while I'm breast feeding. Does this cause some problem?
Most substances you eat or drink (or take orally, as medicine) can pass to your baby in your breast milk. Spicy foods, chocolate and caffeine are just a few things your baby can react to when you ingest them. Be careful about what you eat and drink during breast feeding.

How is caffeine a problem during breast feeding?
Caffeine in breast milk can sometimes cause irritability and sleeplessness in a breast fed baby.

I read an article the other day about a condition called 'insufficient milk syndrome'. What is it?
Insufficient milk syndrome is rare, but it does occur. The baby becomes dehydrated because of breast feeding problems, such as the mother's low milk supply or the baby's failure to drink enough milk.

What kind of problems can insufficient milk syndrome cause?
If it is not detected in the baby and treated, it can cause stroke, blood clot, brain damage and even death of the baby.

How does this syndrome occur?
It can happen when a mother has the idea that breast feeding is the only 'right' method of feeding and takes it to extremes. This woman views using a bottle, even when breast feeding complications occur, as personal failure. It can also happen when a mother is unable to produce enough breast milk, due to genetic defect, injury or breast surgery. However, this problem is very rare.

Your Milk Production

My mother said she couldn't nurse me because she didn't have enough milk. Is this a common problem?
This is *not* a common problem. With some practice and lots of patience, nearly all women can breast feed their babies.

I have a cousin whose breast milk never came in after her triplets were born. Is this common with multiple births?
No, it isn't.

I recently read that I can express my breast milk so my baby can drink it when I'm away from home. How do I do that?
By hand or by using a breast pump that is hand, battery or electrically operated. Expressed milk can be frozen and saved.

How long does it take to express my breast milk?
You'll need 10 to 30 minutes to do this, depending on the method you have, and you'll need to do it one to four times a day (around the time you would normally nurse). You also need a refrigerated place to store the milk and a comfortable, private place where you can relax enough for milk 'let-down' to occur.

How can I store breast milk after it is pumped?
There are several steps you must take to store breast milk safely.

- Pump or express milk into a clean container.
- Label the container with the date and amount of milk collected.
- Freshly pumped breast milk can be kept at room temperature for up to 2 hours, but it's best to refrigerate milk as soon as possible.
- You may store breast milk safely in the refrigerator for up to 72 hours.

I've heard I can freeze breast milk. How do I do that?
For longer storage, you can freeze your breast milk. You can keep it in a refrigerator freezer for 6 months or in a deep freezer (−20°F–29°C) for up to 12 months. Fill the container only three-quarters full to allow for expansion during freezing. Freeze milk in small portions, such as 2–4oz (57–114ml), because these amounts thaw more quickly.

Is it possible to combine fresh breast milk with frozen breast milk?
Yes, this is possible. First, cool breast milk before combining it with previously frozen milk. The amount of thawed breast milk must be more than the amount of fresh breast milk. Never refreeze breast milk!

What's the best way to thaw frozen breast milk?

- Put the container of frozen milk in a bowl of warm water for 30 minutes, or hold container under warm running water.
- *Never* microwave breast milk; it can alter the composition of the milk.
- Swirl the container to blend any fat that might have separated during thawing.
- Feed thawed milk immediately, or store in the refrigerator for up to 24 hours.

The lady at La Leche League told me that if I bottle feed part of the time, my milk supply will be reduced. Is this true?
Yes, it is. Your milk supply is driven by the baby's demand. If you bottle feed part of the time, your baby will not be demanding the breast milk from you, and your body will slow down its production.

Some Common Problems during Breast Feeding

Will it be painful when my milk comes in?

Breast milk becomes more plentiful between 2 and 6 days after birth, when it comes from colostrum to more nourishing mature milk. Your breasts may become engorged and cause you some pain for 24 to 36 hours. Continue breast feeding during this time. Wear a supportive bra, and apply cold compresses to your breasts for short periods. Take paracetamol (Panadol) if pain is severe, but don't take anything stronger.

My friend says she feels a tingling in her breasts when her baby nurses. What causes this?

Soon after a baby begins to nurse, the mother experiences tingling or cramping in her breasts called *milk let-down*, which means milk is flowing into the breast ducts. It occurs several times during feeding. Occasionally a baby will choke a bit when the rush of milk comes too quickly.

I've read that many new mothers have problems with sore nipples. Why?

If you baby doesn't take your nipple into his or her mouth fully during breast feeding, the jaws can compress the nipple and make it sore. But take heart – sore nipples rarely last longer than a couple of days. Continue breast feeding while your breasts are sore.

Is there any other way to prevent sore nipples?

Nipple shields, worn inside your bra between the nipple and fabric, provide some relief. (It keeps tender skin from rubbing on the bra fabric.) A mild cream can also be applied to sore nipples to provide some soothing relief. Ask your pharmacist or doctor for the names of some products that are all right to use during nursing.

My best friend had a very bad breast infection with her last baby. How will I know if I have one?

Large red streaks that extend up to the breast towards the armpit usually indicate a breast infection. If you experience this, call your doctor immediately. An infection can cause a fever to develop within 4–8 hours after the appearance of the red streaks. Antibiotic treatment needs to be started immediately because antibiotics work well only in the first 12–16 hours of infection. Treatment can clear up the infection within 24 hours.

How is a breast infection treated?

If you have a plugged duct, apply a warm compress to the affected area or soak the breast in warm water. Then express milk or breast feed while massaging the tender area. If you develop flu-like symptoms with a sore breast, call your doctor immediately. Antibiotic treatment will be started. You'll also need to rest in bed, and empty the infected breast by pumping or breast feeding every hour or two.

What happens if a breast infection isn't treated?

It can turn into an abscess. This is very painful and may need to be opened and drained.

Is there any way to prevent breast infections?

Yes, there are several things you can do to help prevent an infection.

- Eat correctly, and get enough rest. Doing these two things helps reduce stress and keeps your immune system in top fighting form.
- Don't wear tight-fitting bras – especially underwire-bras – because they block milk flow. This can cause an infection.
- Be sure you empty your breasts regularly. This avoids engorgement.
- After each feeding or pumping, let nipples air-dry for a few minutes.

Should I stop nursing if I get a breast infection?

No, don't stop nursing. It's important to continue breast feeding. If you stop, the infection may get worse.

I recently read that ducts in the breasts can get plugged up. What does this mean?

A plugged milk duct in the breast prevents milk from flowing freely. It results in tender or firm areas of the breast that become more painful after breast feeding. A plugged duct is not red, and you will not have a fever.

How is a plugged duct treated?

It usually takes care of itself if you continue to nurse frequently. Apply warm compresses to the sore area to help with the pain and to open the duct. Paracetamol (Panadol) may also be taken.

If I'm sick, can I still breast feed?

If you have a cold or other virus, it is all right to breast feed. You can breast feed if you're taking an antibiotic, as long as you know the drug is not incompatible with nursing. Ask your doctor or pharmacist if any medicine prescribed for you should not be taken while breast feeding. Be sure to ask *before* you begin taking it.

You should also Know

My breasts are very small. How do I know I'll have enough breast milk?
The size of your breasts doesn't influence the amount of milk you have, so this usually isn't a problem.

I'm embarrassed when I think about breast feeding my baby in public. Is it really acceptable?
In many countries, breast feeding is a natural part of life. In North America, people are more accepting of breast feeding than in the past. My best advice is to gauge each situation separately. If you are comfortable nursing at a friend's house, go ahead. If you feel uncomfortable nursing in a public place, go into the ladies' room or a lounge, and feed there. Look at each instance by itself – you'll soon learn how comfortable you feel feeding your baby away from home.

My sister-in-law said she didn't keep breast feeding her son because he wouldn't settle into a pattern. Is this common?
You may be unprepared for how often your baby will want (and need) to nurse in the first week after birth. You may wonder if it's worth it to continue. Relax and be patient. It will take time for your baby to establish his or her nursing pattern. By the end of the second week, a pattern will probably be established, and your baby will sleep longer between feedings.

Is it all right to substitute bottles for some breast feeding sessions?
It's best to avoid bottles, if possible, for the first month of breast feeding. This is for two reasons – your baby may come to prefer feeding from a bottle (it's not as hard to suck) and your breasts will not produce enough milk.

I don't know how long I'll be able to breast feed my baby because I have to go back to work. Is there a specific period in which it is most important for me to nurse my baby?

Nursing for the first 4 weeks of your baby's life provides the most protection for your baby and the most beneficial hormone release for you to help you recover after the birth. Nursing for the first 6 months is very beneficial for your baby – it provides excellent nutrition and protection against illness. After 6 months, the nutrition and protection aspects are not as critical for your baby. So if you can nurse for only a short period of time, try to stick with it for the first 6 months or at least for the first 4 weeks.

I want to continue breast feeding my baby after I go back to work. Is this possible?

It is possible to continue breast feeding your baby after you return to work. If you breast feed exclusively, you will have to pump your breasts or arrange to see your baby during the day. Or you can nurse your baby at home and provide formula for when you're away.

A friend told me that support at work for her breast feeding seemed to disappear after 4 or 5 months. What can I do about this?

You may have to talk to your employer and co-workers about the situation and attempt to work out a solution that is equitable for everyone.

If I have to be away for a few days, will my breast milk dry up?

You will probably need to pump your breast milk while you are gone. You may be very uncomfortable if you don't because your milk will continue to come in. Take a breast pump with you and discard the breast milk after it is pumped.

I've heard there are special bras to wear while breast feeding. What are they?

Nursing bras are worn for breast feeding. They have cups that open so you can breast feed without having to undress.

When should I buy a nursing bra?

Wait until at least 36 weeks of your pregnancy. If you buy it sooner, it will be very difficult to buy one that fits.

How can I be sure a nursing bra will fit correctly?

Your breasts will become larger when your milk comes in, so buy a bra with at least a finger's width of space between any part of the cup and your breast. Be sure to make allowances for the room taken up by the nursing pads. When trying on the bra, fasten the hooks at their loosest setting. That will make it possible for you to tighten it as your rib cage shrinks after your baby is born.

Are there any other special clothes I should consider for breast feeding?

Yes. Nighties, shift dresses and full-cut blouses have been designed with discreet breast openings so you don't have to get undressed to breast feed. You can reach up inside your outer clothing, unhook your nursing bra and place your baby at your breast without anyone noticing. Draping a light towel or blanket over your shoulder, over the baby's head, adds further coverage.

A few years ago, I had my very small breasts enlarged. Can I breast feed my baby after it is born?

Yes. Many women who have had breast-enlargement surgery are able to breast feed successfully.

Because of back problems caused by extremely large breasts, I had the size of my breasts reduced. Will this affect my ability to breast feed?

You should still be able to breast feed. You may have a decreased production of milk, but usually there is enough.

Someone told me that if I breast feed, my nipples will drip milk when my baby cries. This isn't true, is it?

It is true. This will occur when your baby or any other baby near you, cries. This reflex is called the *milk letdown response* and is normal. To protect your clothing, be sure you wear breast shields.

I'm sure my partner will feel left out if he can't feed the baby. Is there any way he can participate in feeding?

Your partner can help out by getting up at night and bringing the baby to you or by changing the baby. Your partner can also feed your baby expressed breast milk or water.

I know my stepdaughter will want to help me feed the baby, but I'll be nursing. How can I include her?

You can include your stepdaughter by letting her hold or burp the baby after it is fed. If you express your milk, she could feed the baby a bottle of it from time to time.

Should I switch breasts during breast feeding?

Yes, but wait until your baby finishes with one breast before switching to the other one. The consistency of breast milk changes from thinner to richer as the baby nurses. At the next feeding, start your baby on the breast you last nursed with. This will help you keep both breasts stimulated. If your baby only wants to nurse from one breast each feeding, simply switch to the other breast for the next feeding.

If I have any problems breast feeding, what can I do?

Many hospitals have breast feeding specialists you can call for help. Try your doctor – he or she may be able to refer you to someone knowledgeable. You can also look in the telephone book for the *La Leche League*, which is an organisation that promotes breast feeding. Someone from the local group can give you advice and encouragement.

How do I discontinue nursing when my baby is old enough to stop?

You can either taper off gradually or stop at once. Each way has its advantages. If you want to taper off gradually, start offering a bottle every other feeding or offer bottles during the day and nurse at night. If you stop at once, you may have some sleepness nights with a screaming baby, and you may be quite uncomfortable physically with engorged breasts. However, this method takes less time.

At what age (of the baby) do most women stop breast feeding?

That varies from woman to woman. Some women like to nurse until they return to work. Others nurse through the first year. It depends on your situation and your desire.

Glossary

A

abortion – Termination of pregnancy before 20 weeks of pregnancy.

abruptio placentae – See *placental abruption*.

acquired immune deficiency syndrome (Aids) – Debilitating, usually fatal, illness that affects the body's ability to respond to infection. Caused by the human immune deficiency virus (HIV).

aerobic exercise – Exercise that increases your heart rate and causes you to consume oxygen.

afterbirth – see *placenta*.

albuminuria – see *proteinuria*.

alpha-fetoprotein (AFP) – Substance produced by the unborn baby as it grows inside the uterus. Large amounts of AFP are found in amniotic fluid. Larger than normal amounts are found in the maternal bloodstream if neural tube defects are present in the fetus.

alveoli – Ends of the ducts of the lung.

amino acids – Substances that act as building blocks in the developing embryo and fetus.

amniocentesis – Removal of amniotic fluid from the amniotic sac. Fluid is tested for some genetic defects.

amnion – Membrane around the fetus. It surrounds the amniotic cavity.

amniotic fluid – Liquid surrounding the baby inside the amniotic sac.

amniotic sac – Sac that surrounds baby inside the uterus. It contains the baby, the placenta and the amniotic fluid.

ampulla – Dilated opening of a tube or duct.

anaemia – Any condition in which the number of red blood cells is less than normal. Term usually applies to the concentration of the oxygen-transporting material in the blood, which are the red blood cells.

anencephaly – Defective development of the brain combined with the absence of the bones normally surrounding the brain.

angioma – Tumour, usually benign, or swelling composed of lymph and blood vessels.

antenatal cardiolocography – Test in which movements of the baby felt by the mother are recorded along with the changes in the fetal heart rate, to assess well-being of fetus.

antenatal care – Programme of care for a pregnant woman before the birth of her baby.

anti-D immunoglobulin – Substance given during pregnancy and following delivery to prevent isoimmunisation. Also see *Isoimmunisation.*

anti-inflammatory medications – Drugs to relieve pain or inflammation.

Apgar score – Measurement of a baby's response to birth and life on its own. Taken 1 minute and 5 minutes after birth.

areola – Pigmented or coloured ring surrounding the nipple of the breast.

arrhythmia – Irregular or missed heart beat.

aspiration – Swallowing or sucking a foreign body or fluid, such as vomit, into an airway.

asthma – Disease marked by recurrent attacks of shortness of breath and difficulty breathing. Often caused by an allergic reaction.

atonic – Flaccid; relaxed; lacking tone. As in *atonic uterus.*

auto-antibodies – Antibodies that attack parts of your body or your own tissues.

B

beta-sympathomimetics – During pregnancy, they are used to stop labour.

bilirubin – Breakdown product of pigment formed in the liver from haemoglobin during the destruction of red blood cells.

biophysical profile – Method of evaluating a fetus before birth.

biopsy – Removal of a small piece of tissue for microscopic study.

birthing centre – Facility in which a woman labours, delivers and recovers in the same room. It may be part of a hospital, or it may be a freestanding unit.

bloody show – Small amount of vaginal bleeding late in pregnancy; often precedes labour.

Braxton-Hicks contractions – Irregular, painless tightening of uterus during pregnancy.

breech presentation – Abnormal presentation of the fetus. Buttocks or legs come into the birth canal ahead of the head.

C

caesarean section (delivery) – Delivery of a baby through an abdominal incision rather than through the vagina.

candidal vulvovaginitis – Infection caused by yeast or candida. Usually affects the vagina and vulva.

carcinogen – Any cancer-producing substance.

cataract, congenital – Cloudiness of the eye lens present at birth.

cervical smear – Routine screening test that evaluates the presence of premalignant or cancerous conditions of the cervix.

Chadwick's sign – Dark-blue or purple discoloration of the mucosa of the vagina and cervix during pregnancy.

chemotherapy – Treatment of disease by chemical substances or drugs.

chlamydia – Sexually transmitted venereal infection.

chloasma – Extensive brown patches of irregular shape and size on the face or other parts of the body.

chorionic villus sampling (CVS) – Diagnostic test done early in pregnancy. A biopsy of tissue is taken from inside the uterus through the abdomen or the cervical opening to determine abnormalities of pregnancy.

colostrum – Thin, yellow fluid that is the first milk to come from the breast. Most often seen toward the end of pregnancy. It is different in content from milk produced later during nursing.

condyloma acuminatum – Skin tags or warts that are sexually transmitted. Also called *venereal warts*.

congenital problem – Problem present at birth.

conjoined twins – Twins connected at the body; they may share vital organs. Also called *Siamese twins*.

constipation – Bowel movements are infrequent or incomplete.

contraction stress test (CST) – Response of fetus to uterine contractions to evaluate fetal well-being.

crown-to-rump length – Measurement from the top of the baby's head (crown) to the buttocks of the baby (rump).

cystitis – Inflammation of the bladder.

cytomegalovirus (CMV) infection – Infection caused by any of a group of viruses from the herpes virus family.

D

D and C (dilatation and curettage) – Surgical procedure in which the cervix is dilated and the lining of the uterus is scraped.

developmental delay – Condition in which the development of the baby or child is slower than normal.

diabetes, pregnancy-induced – See *gestational diabetes*.

diastasis recti – Separation of abdominal muscles.

dilatation – Expansion of an organ or vessel.

dizygotic twins – Twins derived from two different eggs. Often called *fraternal twins*.

Down's syndrome – Condition in which baby is born mentally retarded and with a generally dwarfed appearance, including a sloping forehead, short, broad hands, a flat nose and low-set ears.

dysplasia – Abnormal, precancerous changes in the cells of the cervix.

dysuria – Difficulty in or pain on urinating.

E

eclampsia – Convulsions and coma in a woman with *pre-eclampsia*. Not related to epilepsy.

ectopic pregnancy – Pregnancy that occurs outside the uterine cavity.

EDC (estimated date of confinement) – Anticipated due date for delivery of the baby. Calculated as 280 days after the first day of the last menstrual period.

effacement – Thinning of cervix.

electronic fetal monitoring – Use of electronic instruments to record the fetal heart beat and the mother's contractions.

embryo – Organism in the early stages of development.

embryonic period – First 10 weeks of gestation (8 weeks of fetal development).

endometrium – Membrane that lines the inside of the uterine wall.

enema – Fluid injected into the rectum for the purpose of clearing out the bowel.

engorgement – Congested; filled with fluid.

epidural block – Type of anaesthesia. Medication is injected around the spinal cord during labour or some types of surgery.

episiotomy – Surgical incision of the vulva (area behind the vagina, above the rectum). Use during delivery to avoid tearing or laceration of the vaginal opening and rectum.

estimated date of confinement – see *EDC*.

external cephalic version (ECV) – Procedure done late in pregnancy in which doctor attempts to move a baby manually from the breech position into the normal head-down position.

F

face presentation – Situation in which baby comes into the birth canal face-first.

fallopian tube – Tube that leads from the cavity of the uterus to the area of the ovary. Also called *uterine tube*.

false labour – Tightening of uterus without dilatation or thinning of the cervix.

fasting blood sugar – Blood test to evaluate the amount of sugar in the blood following a period of fasting.

ferrous gluconate – Iron supplement.

ferrous sulphate – Iron supplement.

fertilisation – Joining of the sperm and egg.

fertilisation age – Dating a pregnancy from the time of fertilisation; 2 weeks earlier than the *gestational age*.

fetal alcohol syndrome (FAS) – Birth defects in an infant born to mother whose alcoholic intake persisted during pregnancy. Infant will have physical abnormalities and mental deficiencies.

fetal anomaly – Fetal malformation or abnormal development.

fetal arrhythmia – See *arrhythmia*.

fetal distress – Problems with the baby that occur before birth or during labour. These endanger the baby and require immediate delivery.

fetal growth retardation – See *intra-uterine growth retardation*.

fetal monitor – Device used before or during labour to listen to and record the fetal heart beat. Can be external monitoring (through maternal abdomen) or internal monitoring (through maternal vagina) of the baby inside the uterus.

fetal period – Time period following the embryonic period until birth.

fetus – Refers to the unborn baby from early pregnancy until birth.

forceps – Special instrument placed around the baby's head, inside the birth canal, to help guide the baby out of the birth canal during delivery.

frank breech – Baby presenting buttocks first. Legs are flexed and knees extended.

fraternal twins – see *dizygotic twins*.

full term baby – Baby born between 38 and 42 weeks of pregnancy.

G

genetic counselling – Consultation between a couple and a specialist about genetic defects and the possibility of presence or recurrence of genetic problems in a pregnancy.

genital herpes simplex – Herpes simplex infection involving the mother's genital area. It can be significant during pregnancy because of the danger to a newborn baby infected with herpes simplex.

gestational age – Dating a pregnancy from the first day of the last menstrual period; 2 weeks longer than fertilisation age. See *fertilisation age*.

gestational diabetes – Occurrence or worsening of diabetes during pregnancy.

globulin – Family of proteins from plasma or serum of the blood.

glucose tolerance test – Blood test done to evaluate the body's response to sugar. Blood is drawn at intervals following ingestion of a sugary substance.

glucosuria – Glucose in the urine.

gonorrhoea – Contagious venereal infection, transmitted primarily by intercourse. Caused by the bacteria *Neisseria gonorrhoea*.

group-B streptococcal infection – Serious infection occurring in the mother's vagina and throat.

H

habitual miscarriage – Occurrence of three or more spontaneous miscarriages.

haematocrit – Measurement of the proportion of blood cells to plasma. Important in diagnosing anaemia.

haemoglobin – Pigment in red blood cell that carries oxygen to body tissues.

haemolytic disease – Destruction of red blood cells. See *Anaemia*.

haemorrhoids – Dilated blood vessels in the rectum or rectal canal.

heartburn – Discomfort or pain that occurs in the chest. Often occurs after eating.

heparin – Substance used to thin the blood.

high-risk pregnancy – Pregnancy with complications that require special medical attention, often from a specialist. Also see *Perinatologist*.

Homan's sign – Pain caused by flexing the toes when a person has a blood clot in the lower leg.

human chorionic gonadotrophin (HCG) – Hormone produced in early pregnancy. Measured in a pregnancy test.

hydramnios – Increased amniotic fluid.

hydrocephalus – Excessive accumulation of fluid around the brain of the baby. Sometimes called *water on the brain*.

hyperbilirubinaemia – Extremely high level of *bilirubin* in the blood.

hyperemesis gravidarum – Severe nausea, dehydration and vomiting during pregnancy. Occurs most frequently during the first trimester. May require brief hospital admission.

hyperglycaemia – Increased blood sugar.

hypertension, pregnancy-induced – High blood pressure that occurs during pregnancy. Defined by an increase in the diastolic or systolic blood pressure.

hyperthyroidism – Elevation of the thyroid hormone in the bloodstream.

hypoplasia – Defective or incomplete development or formation of tissue.

hypotension – Low blood pressure.

hypothyroidism – Low or inadequate levels of thyroid hormone in the bloodstream.

I

identical twins – See *monozygotic twins*.

immune globulin preparation – Substance used to protect against infection with certain diseases, such as hepatitis or measles.

incompetent cervix – Cervix that dilates painlessly, without contractions.

incomplete miscarriage – Miscarriage in which part, but not all, of the uterine contents are expelled.

indigestion – Inability to digest food or difficulty digesting food.

induced labour – Labour started artificially.

inevitable miscarriage – Pregnancy complicated with bleeding and cramping. Results in miscarriage.

insulin – Peptide hormone made by the pancreas. It promotes the use of glucose.

intra-uterine growth retardation (IUGR) – Inadequate growth of the fetus during the last stages of pregnancy. Also called *fetal growth retardation*.

in utero – Within the uterus.

in vitro – Outside the body.

iron-deficiency anaemia – Anaemia produced by lack of iron in the diet. Often seen in pregnancy. Also see *anaemia*.

isoimmunisation – Development of specific antibody directed at the red blood cells of another individual, such as a baby in utero. Often occurs when a rhesus-negative woman carries a rhesus-positive baby or when she is given rhesus-positive blood.

J

jaundice – Yellow staining of the skin, sclera (covering of the eyes) and deeper tissues of the body. Caused by excessive amounts of bilirubin. Treated with phototherapy.

K

ketones – Breakdown product of metabolism found in the blood, particularly in starvation or uncontrolled diabetes.

kidney stone – Small mass or lesion found in the kidney or urinary tract. Can block the flow of urine.

L

labour – The producing dilatation of the cervix to make possible the expelling of a fetus from the uterus.

laparoscopy – Surgical procedure performed for tubal ligation, diagnosis of pelvic pain, diagnosis of ectopic pregnancy and other procedures.

leucorrhoea – Vaginal discharge characterised by a white or yellowish colour. Primarily composed of mucus.

lightening – Dropping or descent of fetus into the pelvis before or during labour.

linea nigra – Line of increased pigmentation running down the abdomen from the belly button to the pubic area during pregnancy.

lochia – Vaginal discharge that occurs after delivery of the baby and placenta.

L/S ratio – Measurement of the relationship of two substances, lecithin and sphingomyelin, in the amniotic fluid. Results give a doctor an indication of the maturity of the baby's lungs.

lupus – See *systemic lupus erythematosus*.

Lyme disease – Infection transmitted to humans by ticks.

M

mammogram – X-ray study of the breasts to identify normal or abnormal breast tissue.

mask of pregnancy – Increased pigmentation over the area of the face under each eye. Commonly has the appearance of a butterfly.

meconium – First intestinal discharge of the newborn; green or yellow in colour. It consists of epithelial or surface cells, mucus and bile. Discharge may occur before or during labour or soon after birth.

melanoma – Pigmented mole or tumour. It may or may not be cancerous.

meningomyelocoele – Congenital defect of the central nervous system of the baby in which membranes and the spinal cord protrude through an opening or defect in the vertebral column.

menstrual age – See *gestational age*.

menstruation – Regular or periodic discharge of a bloody fluid from the uterus.

microcephaly – Abnormally small development of the fetal head.

microphthalmia – Abnormally small eyeballs.

midwife – Nurse who has received extra training in the care of pregnant patients and the delivery of babies.

milk let-down – Tingling or cramping in woman's breast, experienced when breast milk flows into the breast ducts.

miscarriage – End of pregnancy. Giving birth to an embryo or fetus before it can live outside the womb, usually defined as before 20 weeks of pregnancy.

missed abortion – Failed pregnancy, without bleeding or cramping. Sometimes diagnosed by ultrasound weeks or months after a pregnancy fails.

monozygotic twins – Twins conceived from one egg. Often called *identical twins*.

morning sickness – Nausea and vomiting, primarily during the first trimester of pregnancy. Also see *hyperemesis gravidarum*.

mucus plug – Secretions in cervix; often released just before labour.

N

natural childbirth – Labour and delivery in which no medication is used, and the mother remains awake to help deliver the baby. The woman may or may not have taken classes to prepare her for labour and delivery.

neural tube defects – Abnormalities in the development of the spinal cord and brain in a fetus. Also see *anencephaly*; *hydrocephalus*; *spina bifida*.

O

obstetrician – Doctor who specialises in the care of pregnant women and the delivery of babies.

oedema – Swelling of the feet or legs due to water retention.

oligohydramnios – Lack or deficiency of amniotic fluid.

opioids – Synthetic compounds with effects similar to those of opium.

ovarian cycle – Regular production of hormones from the ovary in response to hormonal messages from the brain. The ovarian cycle governs the endometrial cycle.

ovulation – Cyclic production of an egg from the ovary.

ovulatory age – See *fertilisation age*.

oxytocin – Substance that causes uterine contractions; used to induce labour.

P

paediatrician – Doctor who specialises in the care of babies and children.

palmar erythema – Redness of palms of the hands.

paracervical block – Local anaesthetic for cervical dilatation.

perinatologist – Doctor who specialises in the care of high-risk pregnancies.

perineum – Area between the anus and the vagina.

phosphatidyl glycerol – Lipoprotein present in amniotic fluid when fetal lungs are mature.

phospholipids – Fat containing phosphorous compounds. The most important are lecithin and sphingomyelin, which are important in the maturation of fetal lungs before birth.

phototherapy – Treatment of jaundice in a newborn baby. See *jaundice.*

physiological anaemia of pregnancy – Anaemia during pregnancy caused by an increase in the amount of plasma (fluid) in the blood compared to the number of cells in the blood. Also see *anaemia.*

placenta – Organ inside the uterus that is attached to the baby by the umbilical cord. Essential during pregnancy for growth and development of the embryo and fetus. Also called *after-birth* when it is expelled following birth of baby.

placenta praevia – Low attachment of the placenta, very close to or covering the cervix.

placental abruption – Premature separation of the placenta from the uterus.

pneumonitis – Inflammation of the lungs.

polyhydramnios – See *hydramnios.*

post dates birth – Baby born 2 weeks or more past its due date.

postmature baby – Pregnancy of more than 42 weeks' gestation.

postpartum blues – Mild depression after delivery.

postnatal depression – Depression after delivery.

postnatal haemorrhage – Bleeding greater than 18oz (500ml) at time of delivery.

post term baby – See *post dates birth.*

pre-eclampsia – Combination of symptoms significant to pregnancy, including high blood pressure, oedema, swelling and changes in reflexes.

pregnancy diabetes – See *gestational diabetes.*

premature delivery – Delivery before 36 weeks gestation.

prenatal care – Programme of care for a pregnant woman before the birth of her baby.

prepared childbirth – Team used when woman has taken classes to know what to expect during labour and delivery. She may request pain medication if she feels she needs it.

presentation – Term describing which part of the baby comes into the birth canal first.

preterm birth – See *premature delivery*.

propylthiouracil – Medication used to treat thyroid disease.

proteinuria – Protein in urine.

pruritis gravidarum – Itching during pregnancy.

pubic symphysis – Bony prominence in the pelvic bone found in the midline. Landmark from which the doctor often measures during pregnancy to follow growth of the uterus.

pudendal block – Local anaesthesia during labour.

pulmonary embolism – Blood clot from another part of the part of the body that travels to the lungs. Can cause closed passages in the lungs and a decrease in oxygen exchange.

pyelonephritis – Serious kidney infection.

Q

quickening – Feeling the baby move inside the uterus.

R

radiation therapy – Method of treatment for various cancers.

rhesus negative – Absence of *rhesus* antibody in the blood.

rhesus-sensitivity – See *isoimmunisation*.

round ligament pain – Pain caused by stretching of the ligaments on either side of the uterus during pregnancy.

rupture of membranes – Loss of fluid from the amniotic sac. Also called *breaking of waters*.

S

seizure – Sudden onset of a convulsion.

sexually transmitted disease (STD) – Infection which may be transmitted through sexual intercourse.

sickle cell anaemia – Anaemia caused by abnormal red blood cells shaped like a sickle or a cylinder. Occurs most often in black people.

sickle cell trait – Presence of the trait for sickle cell anaemia; not sickle cell disease itself.

sickle crisis – Painful episode caused by sickle cell disease.

skin tag – Flap or extra build up of skin.

sodium – Element found in many foods, particularly salt. Ingestion of too much sodium may cause fluid retention.

spina bifida – Congenital abnormality characterised by a defect in the vertebral column. Membranes of the spinal cord and the spinal cord itself protrude outside the protective bony canal of the spine.

spinal anaesthesia – Anaesthesia given in the spinal canal.

spontaneous miscarriage – Loss of pregnancy during the first 20 weeks of gestation.

stasis – Decreased flow.

station – Estimation of the descent of the baby in the birth canal.

steroids – Drugs of hormone origin used to treat various diseases. Include oestrogen, testosterone, progesterone and prednisolone.

stillbirth – Death of baby before it is born, after 20 weeks of pregnancy.

stress test – Test in which mild contractions of the mother's uterus are induced; fetal heart rate in response to the contractions is noted.

stretch marks – Areas of the skin that are torn or stretched. Often found on the mother's abdomen, breasts, buttocks and legs.

striae gravidarum – See *stretch marks*.

surfactant – Phospholipid present in the lungs that controls surface tension of lungs. Premature babies often lack sufficient amounts of surfactant to breathe without assistance.

syphilis – Sexually transmitted venereal infection caused by *treponema pallidum*.

systemic lupus erythematosus (SLE) – Connective tissue disorder common in women in the reproductive ages. Antibodies made by the person act against person's own tissues.

T

Tay-Sachs disease – Inherited disease characterised by mental and physical retardation, convulsions, enlargement of the head and eventual death. Trait is usually carried by Ashkenazi Jews.

telangiectasia – dilatation or swelling of a small blood vessel. Sometimes called an *angioma*. During pregnancy, another common name is *spider naevi*.

teratogen – A substance that causes abnormal development.

teratology – Branch of science that deals with teratogens and their effects.

thalassaemia – Group of inherited disorders of haemoglobin metabolism, which results in a decrease in the amount of haemoglobin formed. Found most commonly in people of Mediterranean descent.

threatened miscarriage – Bleeding during the first trimester of pregnancy without cramping or contractions.

thrombosis – Formation of a blood clot (thrombus).

thrush – Candida yeast infection occurring in the mouth or mucous membranes of a newborn baby.

thyroid disease – Abnormality of the thyroid gland and its production of thyroid hormone. Also see *hyperthyroidism; hypothyroidism.*

thyroid hormone – Chemical made in the thyroid that affects the entire body.

thyroid panel – Series of blood tests done to evaluate the function of the thyroid gland.

thyroid stimulating hormone (TSH) – Hormone made in the brain that stimulates the thyroid to produce thyroid hormone.

tocolytic agents – Drugs to stop labour.

toxaemia – See *pre-eclampsia.*

toxic streptococcus A – Baterial infection that can cause severe damage; usually starts in a cut on the skin, not as a sore throat, and spreads very quickly. It can involve the entire body.

toxoplasmosis – Infection caused by *toxoplasma gondii.* Can be contracted from handling raw meat or cat faeces.

transverse lie – Situation in which fetus is turned sideways in uterus.

trichomonal vaginitis – Venereal infection caused by trichomonas.

trimester – Method of dividing pregnancy into three equal time periods of about 13 weeks each.

tubal pregnancy – See *ectopic pregnancy.*

U

umbilical cord – Cord that connects the placenta to the developing baby. It removes waste products and carbon dioxide from the baby and brings oxygenated blood and nutrients from the mother through the placenta to the baby.

umbilicus – Belly button.

ureters – Tubes that drain urine from the kidneys to the bladder.

urinary calculi – See *kidney stones.*

uterus – Organ in which an embryo and fetus grow. Also called a *womb.*

V

vaccine – Medication given to patient to cause production of antibodies to protect against subsequent infections.

vacuum extractor – Device used to provide traction on fetal head to aid in delivery.

varicose veins – Blood vessels (veins) that are dilated or enlarged.

vascular spiders – See *telangiectasias*.

vena cava – Major vein in the body that empties into the right atrium of the heart. It returns unoxygenated blood to the heart for transport to the lungs.

venereal warts – See *condyloma acuminatum*.

vernix – Fatty substance made up of epithelial cells that covers fetal skin inside the uterus.

vertex presentation – Head first.

W

womb – See *uterus*.

Y

yeast infection – See *candidal vulvovaginitis; thrush*.

Useful Addresses

Association for Post-Natal Illness (APNI)
25 Jerdan Place
London SW6 1BE
Tel (0171) 386 0868
Network of telephone and postal volunteers who have suffered from postnatal illness and offer information, support and encouragement on a one-to-one basis.

CRY-SIS (East, West and Northern Ireland)
BM CRY-SIS
London WC1N 3XX
Tel (0171) 404 5011
Help and support for parents whose children cry excessively, have a sleep problem or have temper tantrums and other behaviour difficulties. Local voluntary counsellors who have experienced the same difficulties.

Parentline (East and Northern Ireland)
Endway House
The Endway
Hadleigh, Benfleet
Essex SS7 2AN
Tel (01702) 554782
    (01702) 559900 (Helpline)
Voluntary self-help organisation offering confidential support to parents under stress. A network of local telephone helplines is operated by trained parents. Local support groups.

ACAS (Advisory, Conciliation and Arbitration Service) (East, South and West)

Clifton House
83 Euston Road
London NW1 2RB
Tel (0171) 396 5100

Advice on time off for antenatal care and on matters like unfair dismissal. For your nearest office, look in the phone book or ask at your local library or citizens' advice bureau.

Association of Breastfeeding Mothers

26 Holmshaw Close
London SE26 4TH
Tel (0181) 778 4769

Telephone advice service for breast feeding mothers and those wanting to breast feed. Runs support groups (babies welcome). Help given to those wishing to set up a group in their area.

Association for Improvements in the Maternity Services (AIMS)

40 Kingswood Avenue
London NW6 6LS
Tel (0181) 960 5585
or
40 Leamington Terrace
Edinburgh EH10 4JL
Tel (0131) 229 6259

Voluntary pressure group which aims for improvements in maternity services. Support and advice about parents' rights, complaints procedures and choices within maternity care, including home birth.

Caesarean Support Network

c/o Sheila Tunstall
2 Hurst Park Drive
Liverpool L36 1TF
Tel (0151) 480 1184

Offers emotional support and practical advice to mothers who have had or may need a caesarean delivery. Can put you in touch with a local mother who has undergone a caesarean section and understands the problems.

Citizens' Advice Bureaux (CABs)

Information and advice on topics including benefits, maternity rights, debts, housing, consumer, employment and legal problems as well as family and personal difficulties. Have details of useful national and local organisations. Free and confidential. Opening times vary. Ask for the address at your local library or look in the phone book.

Community Health Councils (CHCs)

(Local Health Councils in Scotland; local Health and Social Services Councils in Northern Ireland)

Represent the interests of consumers in the NHS. Can advise you on local NHS services and your entitlements and help you if you are having difficulties or wish to make a complaint. Have information on other local organisations. Look in the phone book under your health authority/health board/local Health and Social Services Board.

Family Health Services Authorities (FHSAs)

These have replaced Family Practitioner Committees. If you're new to an area they can give you a list of local doctors including those with a special interest in pregnancy and childbirth. If you are having difficulty in finding a general practitioner to take you on, contact the FHSA. Look in the phone book under the name of your local health authority health board. Contact your local Health and Social Services Board or

Central Services Agency for Health and Personal Social Services (CSA)

25 Adelaide Street
Belfast BT2 8FH
Tel (01232) 324431

Independent Midwives Association

Nightingale Cottage
Shamblehurst Lane
Botley Hampshire SO32 2BY

Free advice to women thinking about a home birth. Offers full care to women who book with them for home births. They also have their own birthing centres. Fees vary. Send an A5 sae for information.

La Leche League (Great Britain)
BM 3424
London WC1N 3XX
Tel (0171) 242 1278
Help and information for women wanting to breast feed their babies and personal counselling to mothers having problems in breast feeding. Local groups hold friendly, informal discussions on breast feeding, birth and parenthood.

Labour Relations Agency (Northern Ireland)
Windsor House
9–15 Bedford Street
Belfast BT2 7NU
Tel (01232) 321442
Advice on maternity rights in Northern Ireland.

Maternity Alliance
45 Beech Street
London EC2P 2LX
Tel (0171) 588 8582
Information on all aspects of maternity services, rights at work and benefits for families.

National Association for Maternal and Child Welfare
1st Floor, 40–42 Osnaburgh Street
London NW1 3ND
Tel (0171) 383 4115
Telephone advice on childcare and family life.

National Childbirth Trust (NCT)
Alexandra House
Oldham Terrace
London W3 6NH
Tel (0181) 992 8637
National charity with branches throughout the UK. Runs antenatal classes giving information on labour and practice of relaxation, breathing, massage and active positions for labour and birth. Has breast feeding counsellors who will help with feeding. Also offers postnatal support from other mothers and runs postnatal exercise classes in some areas. Provides information for parents with disabilities or medical conditions and puts them in touch with each other. Local branches.

Gingerbread
49 Wellington Street
London WC2E 7BB
Tel (0171) 240 0953
Self-help associations for one-parent families. A network of local groups offers mutual support, friendship, information, advice and practical help. Do get in touch if you are pregnant and on your own.
Gingerbread Northern Ireland
169 University Street
Belfast BT7 1HR
Tel (01232) 231417
Gingerbread Wales
Room 16
Albion Chambers
Cambrian Place
Swansea
West Glamorgan SA1 1RN
Tel (01792) 648728

MAMA (Meet-a-Mum Association)
c/o Briony Hallam
14 Willis Road
Croydon CR0 2XX
Tel (0181) 665 0357
Support for mothers suffering from postnatal depression or who feel lonely and isolated looking after a child at home. Will try to put you in touch with another mother who has experienced similar problems, or with a group of mothers locally, or help you to find ways of meeting people.

National Council for One Parent Families (East, West and Northern Ireland)
255 Kentish Town Road
London NW5 2LX
Tel (0171) 267 1361
and
One Parent Families Scotland
13 Gayfield Square
Edinburgh EH1 3NX
Tel (0131) 556 3899
Information on benefits and employment rights in pregnancy, social security, taxation, housing problems and maintenance.

Illness and Disability

Compassionate Friends
53 North Street
Bristol BS3 1EN
Tel (0117) 953 9639
An organisation of and for bereaved parents. Advice and support. Local Groups.

Foundation for the Study of Infant Deaths (Cot Death Research and Support) (East, West and Northern Ireland)
14 Halkin Street
London SW1X 7DP
Tel (0171) 235 0965
Support and information for parents bereaved by a sudden infant death and support with any subsequent babies. Can put parents in touch with local support groups of other parents who have also suffered bereavement. Produce infant care guidance card including symptoms of serious illness to watch out for in babies.
In Northern Ireland:
Friends of the Foundation for the Study of Infant Deaths
7 Glenaan Avenue
Belfast BT17 9AT
Tel (01232) 622688

Miscarriage Association
c/o Clayton Hospital
Northgate
Wakefield
West Yorks WF1 3JS
Tel (01924) 200799
Information, advice and support for women who have had, or who are having, a miscarriage. Local contact groups.

SATFA (Support around Termination or Abnormality) (East, West and Northern Ireland)
73–75 Charlotte Street
London WIP 1LB
Tel (0171) 631 0285
Registered charity offering support and information to parents who are concerned about antenatal testing, or are faced with the decision of whether to terminate a pregnancy following the diagnosis of abnormality in their unborn baby. Ongoing support given to parents who decide to terminate pregnancy. Network of local contact groups sharing similar experiences.

Stillbirth and Neonatal Death Society (SANDS)
28 Portland Place
London W1N 4DE
Tel (0171) 436 5881
Information and a national network of support groups for bereaved parents.

BLISS
17–21 Emerald Street
London WC1N 3QL
Tel (0171) 831 9393
Parent support network providing emotional and practical support to the families of babies who need intensive or special care. Local groups.

Contact a Family
170 Tottenham Court Road
London W1P 0HA
Tel (0171) 383 3555
National charity offering information, advice and support to parents of children with special needs and disabilities. Links parents to local support groups for general support or to nationally run groups, or, in the case of rare disorders, to individuals in similar circumstances.

Genetic Interest Group (GIG)
Farringdon Point
29–35 Farringdon Road
London EC1M 3JB
Tel (0171) 430 0090
Umbrella body for support groups working with those affected by specific genetic disorders. Provides information for individuals at risk and their families about services available within the NHS and elsewhere. Can put you in touch with the relevant support group.

Association for Spina Bifida and Hydrocephalus (ASBAH) (East and West)
ASBAH House
42 Park Road
Peterborough PE1 2UQ
Tel (01733) 555988
In Scotland:
Scottish Spina Bifida Association
190 Queensferry Road
Edinburgh EH4 2BW
Tel (0131) 32 0743
In Northern Ireland:
Northern Ireland Spina Bifida and Hydrocephalus Association
73 New Row
Coleraine BT52 1EJ
Tel (01265) 515222
Information, advice, counselling and support for parents. Local support groups.

Cleft Lip Palate Association (CLAPA)
1 Eastwood Gardens
Kenton
Newcastle-upon-Tyne NE3 3DQ
Tel (0191) 285 9396
Voluntary organisation of parents and professionals offering support to families of babies born with cleft lip and/or palate. Feeding equipment available. Local groups.

Cystic Fibrosis Trust
Alexandra House
5 Blyth Road
Bromley BR1 3RS
Tel (0181) 464 7211
In Northern Ireland:
Cystic Fibrosis Trust in Northern Ireland
20 Bryansburn Road
Bangor
Co Down BT20 3SB
Tel (01247) 272781
In Wales:
Cystic Fibrosis Trust in Wales
18 Pine Tree Close
Radyr
Cardiff CF4 8RQ
Tel (01222) 843394
Information and support for parents of children with cystic fibrosis and for people worried about the possibility of passing on the illness. Local groups.

Down's Syndrome Association (East and West)
155 Mitcham Road
Tooting, London SW17 9PG
Tel (0181) 682 4001
In Scotland:
Scottish Down's Syndrome Association
159–160 Balgreen Road
Edinburgh EH11 3AU
Tel (0131) 313 4225
In Northern Ireland:
Down's Syndrome Association
2nd Floor
Bryson House
28 Bedford Street
Belfast BT2 7FE
Tel (01232) 243266
Information, advice, counselling and support for parents of children with Down's syndrome. Local groups. 24-hour helpline.

Haemophilia Society
123 Westminster Bridge Road
London SE1 7HR
Tel (0171) 928 2020
In Northern Ireland:
Haemophilia Society
67 Woodvale Road
Belfast BT13 3BN
Tel (01232) 740001
*Information, advice and practical help for families affected by haemophilia.
Some local groups.*

Jennifer Trust for Spinal Muscular Atrophy
11 Ash Tree Close
Wellesbourne
Warwickshire CV35 9SA
Tel (01789) 842377
*Self-help group offering information and support to parents of children with
the disease. Can put you in touch with other parents. Equipment on loan.*

**MENCAP (Royal Society for Mentally Handicapped Children and
Adults) (East, West and Northern Ireland)**
MENCAP National Centre
123 Golden Lane
London EC1Y 0RT
Tel (0171) 44 0454
In Scotland:
ENABLE (Scotland)
6th Floor
7 Buchanan Street
Glasgow G1 3HL
Tel (0141) 226 4541
In Northern Ireland:
MENCAP in Northern Ireland
4 Annadale Avenue
Belfast BT7 3JH
Tel (01232) 691351

In Wales:

MENCAP in Wales
169 City Road
Cardiff CF2 3JB
Tel (01222) 494933
Information, support and advice for parents of children with mental handicap. Local groups

Muscular Dystrophy Group of Great Britain and Northern Ireland
7–11 Prescott Place
London SW3 6BS
Tel (0171) 720 8055
Information, advice and support for families affected by muscular dystrophy.

National Society for Phenylketonuria and Allied Disorders
7 Southfield Close
Willen
Milton Keynes MK15 9LL
Tel (01908) 691653
Self-help organisation offering information and support to families affected by the disorder. Newsletter.

Northern Ireland Council for Orthopaedic Development (NICOD)
Malcolm Sinclair House
31 Ulsterville Avenue
Belfast BT9 7AS
Tel (01232) 666188
Offers advice and support to parents of children with cerebral palsy.

REACH (The Association for Children with Hand or Arm Deficiency)
12 Wilson Way
Earls Barton
Northamptonshire NN6 0NZ
Tel (01604) 811041
Information and support to parents of children with hand or arm problems. Can put you in touch with individual families in a similar situation or local groups.

SENSE (National Deaf, Blind and Rubella Association)
11–13 Clifton Terrace
London N4 3SR
Tel (0171) 272 7774
In Northern Ireland:
SENSE (National Deaf, Blind and Rubella Association)
Wilton House
5 College Square North
Belfast BT1 6AR
Tel (01232) 705858
Information, advice and support for families of deaf, blind and rubella handicapped children.

Sickle Cell Society
54 Station Road
Harlesden
London NW10 4UA
Tel (0181) 961 7795/8346
Information, advice and counselling on sickle cell disease.

Society for Mucopolysaccharide Diseases
55 Hill Avenue
Amersham
Buckinghamshire HP6 5BX
Tel (01494) 434156/762789
Information and support to families of children affected by this and related disorders. Local groups.

SCOPE
12 Park Crescent
London W1N 4EQ
Tel (0171) 636 5020
In Wales:
SCOPE
3 Links Court
Links Business Park
St Mellons
Cardiff CF3 0SP
Tel (01222) 797706
Offers advice and support to parents of children with cerebral palsy.

Tay-Sachs and Allied Diseases Association
c/o Royal Manchester Children's Hospital
Pendlebury
Manchester M27 4HA
Tel (0161) 794 4696 ext 2384
Screening for carrier status before and during pregnancy. Information, counselling and practical support to families affected by these disorders.

Toxoplasmosis Trust
Room 26
61–71 Collier Street
London N1 9BE
Tel (0171) 713 0599
Information, counselling and advice for pregnant women with toxoplasmosis, parents of infected children and others with toxoplasmosis.

The UK Thalassaemia Society
107 Nightingale Lane
London N8 7QY
Tel (0181) 348 0437
Information, advice and support for families affected by thalassaemia and for possible carriers.

Resources for Parents of Multiple Pregnancies

The Multiple Births Foundation
Queen Charlotte's and Chelsea Hospital
Goldhawk Road
London W6 0XG
Tel (0181) 740 3519
Fax (0181) 740 3041
or
Lansdowne Health Centre
Winson Green
Birmingham B18 7EE
Tel (0121) 554 3801 ext. 4056
or

The Children's Centre
The District Hospital
Wigginton Road
York YO2 2LD
Tel (01904) 632 990

Twins and Multiple Births Association (TAMBA)
PO Box 30
Little Sutton
South Wirral L66 1TH
Tel (0151) 348 0020
Twinline (Helpline) (01732) 868 000
In Northern Ireland:
PO Box 342
Belfast BT5 5PQ
Tel (01232) 791 327

Cleveland Twins Centre
c/o Cleveland Multiple Births Trust
2 Buttermore Road
Redcar
Cleveland TS10 1LN
Tel (01642) 450 400

Index

Page numbers in *italic* indicate an entry in the glossary.

abdomen
    itching 134
    pain 16, 176, 178
    skin after pregnancy 254
abortion 61, *283*
    rhesus negativity 39
    spontaneous 178
accidents 176
Accutane 76
acne
    mothers-to-be 76, 205
    newborns 261
acyclovir 160
aerobic exercise *283*
    during pregnancy 94
after-baby blues 254
afterbirth *see* placenta
after pregnancy 249–82
    birth control 256–7
    feeding 269–82
    home safety 257
    newborns 258–68
    postnatal check ups 255–6
    recovery 251–5
age *see* older mothers-to-be; older
    partners
Aids (acquired immune deficiency
    syndrome) 17, 162–3, *283*
    drug use 169
    tests 4, 162–3
air embolus 209
air pollution 123
alcohol use

before pregnancy 3, 16
during breast feeding 273
during pregnancy 127, 166–7, 179,
    191
partner's 154
alcoholism 73
allergies
    during pregnancy 37–8
    milk 273
alpha-fetoprotein (AFP) *283*
    test 23, 51, 59–60, 71, 211
alveoli *283*
aminopterin 75
amitriptyline 137
amnio acids *283*
amniocentesis 56–9, 71, 211, *283*
    compared with chorionic villus
        sampling 61
    older mothers-to-be 14, 49, 56
    rhesus negativity 39
    ultrasound scan before 54, 57
amnion *283*
amniotic fluid 6, *283*
    fetal swallowing 121, 125
    measuring 54
    meconium 125–6
    see also amniotic fluid; breaking of
        waters
amniotic sac 6–7, 188, *283*
amphetamines 168
ampulla 6, *283*
anaemia 43–5, *283*
    causing dizziness 40
    fatigue 99
    fetal 32, 168
    intra-uterine growth retardation 127

iron supplements 10, 88
  megaloblastic 73
  multiple pregnancies 112
  newborns 259
  see also sickle cell anaemia
anaesthesia
  during labour 222, 230–3
  tubal litigation 252
analgesia 230
androgens 75
anencephaly 60, *283*
  detecting 58
angel dust 169
angioma 133, *284*
antacids 36
antenatal cardiolocography *284*
antenatal care 22–3, *284*
  accompanied 153, 207–8
antenatal classes 114, 203–4
antenatal vitamins 44, 72–3, 87–8
antibiotics
  breast feeding 278–9
  breast infections 277, 278
  dental problems 142
anti-coagulants 75
anti-convulsants 167
anti-depressants 137, 167
anti-D immunoglobulin 39, 51, 181, *284*
anti-inflammatory medications *284*
anti-seizure medicines 188
anxiety in partners 153
Apgar scores 242, 259, *284*
appendicitis 63
areola 144, *284*
arrhythmia 120–1, *284*
artificial sweeteners 84–5
aspartame 84
aspiration *284*
aspirin 76, 77
asthma *284*
  before pregnancy 9
  during pregnancy 46
atonic *284*
auto-antibodies *284*
AZT 163

babies *see* newborns
baby-proofing a house 257

backache 148, 194
back pain 48, 95, 191, 195, 253
back problems, tests before pregnancy 11
bag of waters 7, 188
barbiturates 167, 168
bathing during pregnancy 205
bed rest 177, 217–18
before pregnancy 1–17
  alcohol use 166
  birth control 8
  exercise 15–16
  health 8–12, 21
  nutrition 14–15
  preparing for pregnancy 3–4
  sexually transmitted diseases 17
  working 17
benefits 107–8
benzodiazepine 167, 168
beta-sympathomimetics 218, *284*
bilirubin 263, *284*
biophysical profile 71, 68–9, 71, 244,
  284
biopsy 64, *284*
birth canal 7
birth control
  after pregnancy 256–7
  before pregnancy 8
  effects on fetus 77–8
birth control pill *see* oral contraceptives
birth defects (congenital problems)
  barbiturate use 168
  chances of 122
  cocaine use 170
  excessive vitamin intake 12, 73
  family history 57
  genetic counselling 13
  maternal epilepsy 10
  opioid use 169
  partner's exposure to chemicals 154
  tranquilliser use 168
  workplace hazards 104
birthing centre *284*
bladder infections 11, 41, 42, 143
bleeding
  gums 141
  nose 38
  see also vaginal bleeding
blood clots 184–6

blood counts 23, 51
blood pressure *see* hypertension;
    hypotension
blood sugar 41
    test 23
    see also hyperglycaemia;
        hypoglycaemia
blood tests 181
    alpha-fetoprotein 23, 59–60, 71,
        211
    fetal 69–70, 228–9
    newborns 259
    quantitative HCG 50
blood transfusions 39, 43
blood typing 4, 23, 51
bloody show 224, 225, *284*
bodily changes during pregnancy 5,
    129–48
bonding 273
    by partners 153–4
bone tumours 47
bottle feeding 271–2
    sleep patterns 266
bowel movements after delivery 227
brain damage 34
Braxton-Hicks contractions 138, 215,
    284
breaking of waters (rupture of
    membranes) 7, 188–9, 215–16
    after a fall 178
    bathing after 205
    premature 217
    sexual activity after 151
breast cancer 11, 47, 186
breast feeding 270, 272–82
    birth control 256, 257
    breast cancer 47
    dieting 254
    nursing bras 197
    sleep patterns 266
    triplets 115
    twins 114
breast milk 270, 275–6
    stopping the flow 252
breasts
    changes during pregnancy 5, 21,
        144–6
    infections 277–8

lumps 186
    pain after birth 253
    regaining normal size 254
    size, and breast feeding 279
    soreness 144, 206
breast shells 146
breathing exercises 100
breathlessness during exercise 16, 93, 95
breech presentation 112, 238–9, *284*
Brufen 76
burping 270

caesarean sections 48, 233–7, 240, *285*
    breech presentation 239
    herpes 160
    intra-uterine growth retardation
        127
    multiple pregnancies 114, 233
    older mothers-to-be 14, 48
    placenta praevia 190, 233
    placental abruption 191, 233
    premature labour 218
    recovery 251
caffeine 37, 86–7, 167
    breast feeding 273, 274
    and infertility 12
    in medicines 12, 76, 86–7
calcium 142
cancer 46–7
    breast 11, 47, 186
    childhood 104, 154
Candarel 84
candidal vulvovaginitis 157–8, *285*
carbohydrate intake 81
carcinogens *285*
cardiotocograms 65, 71, 244
cardiovascular defects 168
car seats 219–20, 257, 268
CAT (computerised tomographic) scans
    11, 63
cataracts, congenital 34, 123, *285*
cats
    accepting the baby 207
    toxoplasmosis 31
centre of gravity, changing 148
cerebral palsy 28, 33, 34
cervical cultures 23, 51
cervical smears 4, 22, 51, 64, *285*

cervix 7
  see also dilatation; effacement;
    incompetent cervix
Chadwick's sign 144, *285*
chemotherapeutic drugs 75
chemotherapy 48, *285*
chicken pox 32, 34
children at antenatal clinics 208
chiropractors 48
chlamydia 17, 161, *285*
chloasma 133, *285*
chlordane 35
cholesterol 85
chorionic villus sampling (CVS) 59,
    60–1, 71, *285*
  Down's syndrome 60, 211
  older mothers-to-be 14
chromosomal abnormalities
  miscarriage 178
  older couples 14
chronic medical problems 8, 22
climbing 102, 252
cloth nappies 267
CMV *see* cytomegalovirus
cocaine 16, 169–70
Codafen 76
codeine 169
coil *see* IUCDs
cold remedies 167
colic 264–5
colostrum 145, 282, *285*
colposcopy 64
complete breech presentation 239
computer terminals 103
computerised tomograph scans (CAT
    scans, CT scans) 11, 63
condoms 17, 78
condyloma acuminatum (condylomata,
    genital warts, venereal warts) 17,
    158–60, *285*
congenital problems *285 see also* birth
    defects
conjoined (Siamese) twins 112, *285*
conjunctivitis 162
constipation 83, 88, 140–1, *285*
contact lenses 219
contact sports 15, 94
contraception *see* birth control

contraction stress test (CST) 65, 66, 69,
    285
contractions 222, 223
  accompanied by bleeding 137
  Braxton-Hicks 138, 215, *284*
  home monitoring 64–5
  sexual activity 151
  timing 225–6
Coombs' test 259
cot death *see* sudden infant death
    syndrome
cots 257
cough medicines 76, 167
couvade 154
crack cocaine 170
cramping 180
cravings 84
Crohn's disease 73
crown-to-rump length 118, 119, *285*
CT (computerised tomographic) scans
    11, 63
CVS *see* chorionic villus sampling
cycling 94
  stationary 94, 194
cystic fibrosis 60, 71
cystinuria 58
cystitis 143, *285*
cytomegalovirus (CMV) 31–2, 34, 104,
    123, *285*
cytotoxic drugs 104

dairy products 82
D and C (dilation and curettage) 181,
    192, *285*
DDT exposure 35
decongestants 38
deep vein thrombosis 184–5
dehydration 263
delivery 240–1
  benefits of exercise 94
  multiple pregnancies 114
  partner's involvement 156
  of the placenta 209
dental care 141–2
  after morning sickness 26, 142
dental X-rays 63, 142
depression 74, 137
  after-baby blues 254

desipramine 137
developmental delay *285*
  maternal phenylketonuria 84
  workplace hazards 104
dexamethasone 70
diabetes
  before pregnancy 3, 4, 8, 9
  caesarean sections 236
  during pregnancy 41, 45–6, 68, 140
  family history 22
  older mothers-to-be 13, 14
diarrhoea
    during pregnancy 31
    newborns 263
diastasis recti 147, *286*
dieting
  after pregnancy 254
  during breast feeding 274
  during pregnancy 15
Diflucan 158
dilatation 7, 221, *286*
  during labour 222, 223, 224
  monitoring 66–7
diphtheria vaccination 79
disposable nappies 267
dizygotic twins 110, *286*
dizziness 40–1, 43
  during exercise 16, 95
doctors
  choosing baby's 198–9
  choosing mother-to-be's 23–5
  starting visits early 4, 21, 50
  when to call 176, 262
dogs 206–7
donor insemination 173, 174
doppler ultrasound 62, 120
douching 144, 209
Down's syndrome 58–9, 211, *286*
  detecting 54, 57, 59, 60, 71, 211
  genetic counselling 13
  older mothers-to-be 14, 48, 49
  older partners 14, 155
drinking (alcohol) *see* alcohol use
drinking (water) *see* water, drinking
driving during pregnancy 201–2
dropping *see* lightening
drug use
  and alcohol use 167

before pregnancy 3, 16
  during pregnancy 127, 167–70
  by partners 154, 155
drugs for premature labour 218
due dates 116, 193
  ultrasound scans 53, 54
dysplasia *286*
dysuria *286*

ears
  cleaning 267
  infections 262
  see also hearing
eating
  to alleviate heartburn 36
  to alleviate morning sickness 25–6
  and blood sugar 41
  cravings 84
  during breast feeding 274
  during diarrhoea attacks 31
  during labour 226, 227
  eating out 86
  exercise 94
  late-night snacks 85
  see also nutrition
eclampsia 187, *286*
ectopic pregnancy 7, 182–4, *286*
  identifying 54
  IUCDs 77, 182
  pelvic inflammatory disease 161, 182
  rhesus negativity 39
EDC (estimated date of confinement)
  286
effacement 7, *286*
  monitoring 66
electric blankets 210
electrolysis 209
electrolyte solution 263
electronic fetal monitoring *286*
ELISA test 162
embarrassment
  breast feeding 279
  when questioning doctors 25
embryo 6, *286*
  difference from fetus 117
embryonic period 122, *286*
emergency childbirth 244–7
emotions 195

changes 136–7
single mothers-to-be 172
employment *see* working
endocarditis 169
endometrium 286
enemas 227, 286
engorgement 286
environmental hazards 33, 35
    partner's exposure 154
Epanutin 46, 75
epidural block 220, 222, 231–2, 286
epilepsy
    before pregnancy 10
    during pregnancy 46
    folic acid supplements 10, 73
episiotomy 224, 227, 237–8, 286
    checking 251
    infections 252
equal-parenthood partnership 155, 235
ergometrine 222, 224, 242
erythroblastosis fetalis 58
erythromycin 161
estimated date of confinement *see* EDC
ethylene oxide 104
exercise
    after pregnancy 254
    before pregnancy 3, 15–16
    during pregnancy 90–5, 136
    legs and feet 102
    multiple pregnancies 113
    to relieve stress 100
expressing milk 275
extended maternity absence 106
external cephalic version 239–40, 286
external fetal monitoring 68, 228
eyes
    abnormalities 75
    conjunctivitis 162
    drops 242, 260
    gooey 266
    infections 161
    microphthalmia 123
    opening in fetus 122
    problems 32
    puffiness 260
    sight loss 28
    squinting 261
    wandering 261

see also cataracts, congenital;
    microphthalmia

face presentation 239, 286
facial hair 147, 209
faintness 95
fallopian tubes 6, 7, 287
falls during pregnancy 177–8
false labour 221, 287
families
    disapproval of single mothers-to-be
        172
    support 115, 173
family practitioners 23
fasting blood sugar 45, 287
fat intake 81, 83–4
fathers *see* partners
fatigue
    after pregnancy 253
    during pregnancy 21, 99–100
    older mothers-to-be 49
feeding 269–82
feet
    exercises 102
    swelling 5, 102, 194
Fenbid 76
ferning test 189
ferrous gluconate 287
ferrous sulphate 287
fertilisation 6, 287
fertilisation age (ovulatory age) 116,
    193, 287
fertility drugs 109
fetal alcohol syndrome (FAS) 154, 166,
    167, 287
fetal anomalies 122–3, 287
    cancer treatments 47
    detecting 58, 59
    folate deficiency 73
    multiple pregnancies 111
    premature labour 217
    rubella 51
fetal blood sampling 68–70, 228–9
fetal death
    cancer treatments 47
    intra-uterine growth retardation
        126–7
    Lyme disease 29

multiple pregnancies 111
premature labour 217
smoking 165
syphilis 34
fetal distress 126, 127, 233, 287
fetal growth retardation *see* intra-
uterine growth retardation
fetal monitoring 67–8, 228, 287
fetal period 287
fetoscopy 62
fetus *287*
changes whilst growing 116–28
difference from embryo 117
effects of Aids 162, 163
effects of diabetes 45
effects of drug use 16, 168, 169, 170
effects of environmental poisons 33,
35
effects of maternal health 21, 26–33,
34
effects of medicines 75, 123
effects of sexual activity 149
effects of sexually transmitted diseases
157, 159, 161
effects of urinary tract infections 143
heartbeat 62, 67–8, 90, 119–21, 228
movement 138–40
risks from X-rays 63
testing 68–71
fevers, mothers-to-be 27, 176
fibre, dietary 83, 141
floating 140
fluconazole 158
fluid intake 85–6
to alleviate asthma 46
during breast feeding 274
during diarrhoea attacks 31
during urinary tract infections 143
fluoride supplements 88
fluoxetine 74
flying during pregnancy 199–200
folic acid
in leafy vegetable 83
and smoking 165
folic acid supplements 73
before pregnancy 12
epilepsy 10, 73
placental abruption 191

food *see* eating; nutrition
forceps 231, 241, *287*
formula 272
frank breech presentation 239, *287*
fraternal twins 110
freezing breast milk 276
fruit in diet 83
full term babies 118, *287*

gas and air 224
gastrointestinal defects 59
Gaviscon 36, 77
Gelusil 36, 77
general anaesthesia 23
general practitioners 23
genetic abnormalities 60, 71, 179
genetic counselling 13, 51–2, *287*
genetic screening 179
genital herpes simplex 17, 160–1, *287*
genital infections 179
see also sexually transmitted diseases
genital warts *see* condyloma acuminatum
German measles *see* rubella
gestational age (menstrual age) 116,
193, *288*
gestational diabetes *288*
globulin 288
glucose tolerance test 45, 51, *287*
glucosuria 46, *288*
gonadotrophin 110
gonorrhoea 17, 161–2, *288*
group-B streptococcal infection 28–9,
34, *288*
growth retardation 75, 111, 166
see also intra-uterine growth
retardation
gums
bleeding 141
nodules 141
gynaecological cancers 47

habitual miscarriage 13, 51, 92, 180, *288*
haematocrit *288*
haemoglobin *288*
haemolytic disease *288*
haemophilia 58
haemorrhoids 36–7, *288*
hair

changes during pregnancy 5, 146
dying and permanent waving 206
facial 147, 209
newborns 260
hallucinogens 169
hashish (marijuana) 16, 168
hazardous substances 103, 155
HCG *see* human chorionic
   gonadotrophin
head
   fetal growth 119
   shape, newborns 260
   size, newborns 260
headaches 37, 176
health
   before pregnancy 8–12
   during pregnancy 21–49
   newborns 262–3
   workplace 107
hearing
   fetal 122
   loss 28, 34, 75
   newborns 122
heart, fetal
   defects 32, 34, 45, 58–9, 123
   disease 75
heart, mothers-to-be
   disease 92
   palpitations 95
   problems 9–10
heartbeat, fetal 119–21
   hearing 62, 120
   maternal exercise 90
   monitoring 67–8, 228
heartburn 5, 35–6, 113, 288
heart rate, mothers-to-be 15, 91–2
heparin 185, 288
hepatitis 27–8, 34
   and drug use 169
   tests 4, 23, 51
   vaccination, newborns 242
heptachlor 35
herbal preparations 12
herbal wraps 210
heroin 169
herpes 17, 160–1
   fetal 58
   sexual activity 151, 161

herpes-zoster 32
high blood pressure *see* hypertension
high risk pregnancies 54, 200, *288*
HIV 17, 162–3
Homan's sign *288*
home delivery, emergency 245
home safety 257
home uterine monitoring 64–5
hospital 218–20
   during pregnancy 26
   length of stay 251
   premature babies 124, 202
   private care 202
   specialised 24
human chorionic gonadotrophin (HCG)
   7, *288*
human papillomavirus (HPV) 159
husbands *see* partners
hydramnios 112, 217, *288*
hydrocephalus 54, 124–5, *288*
hydroxyurea 11
hyperbilirubinaemia 263, *288*
hyperemesis gravidarum 25, *288*
hyperglycaemia 41, 45, *289*
hypertension 40
   caesarean sections 236
   cocaine use 169
   exercise 92
   older mothers-to-be 13, 14, 48
   possible effects of 9, 127, 190, 217
   pre-eclampsia 186, 187
   pregnancy-induced 41, 65, *289*
hyperthyroidism *289*
hypoallergenic protein formula 272
hypoglycaemia 41
hypoplasia *289*
hypotension 40–1, *289*
hypothyroidism 75, 259, *289*
hysterectomy 192

ibuprofen 76
identical twins 110
immune globulin preparation *289*
immunisation 78–9
incapacity benefit 108
incompetent cervix 40, *289*
   exercise 92
   premature labour 217

prolonged standing 17
  sexual activity 151
incomplete breech presentation 239
incomplete miscarriage 180, 289
indigestion 5, 36, 289
induced labour 216, 244, 289
inevitable miscarriage 180, 289
infant mortality 160, 165
infections
  breaking of waters 216
  effects on fetus 27
  fetal 127
  home uterine monitoring 65
  miscarriage 179
  newborns 162
infertility, links with caffeine 12
injury during pregnancy 176
insufficient milk syndrome 275
insulin 9, 289
insurance 4
  private health 203
internal fetal monitoring 67, 228
intestinal blockage 59
intrathecal anaesthesia 232
intra-uterine growth retardation (IUGR)
    126–7, 289
  alcohol use 166, 167
  anaemia 44
  cancer treatments 47
  drug use 168, 169
  evaluating 68
  hypertension 9
  medicines 75
  multiple pregnancies 111
  PCBs 35
  pesticides 35
intravenous drips 220
intravenous feeding 25, 26
intravenous fluids 226
in utero 289
inverted nipples 145–6
in vitro 289
in vitro fertilisation 111, 179
iodine 75
ionizing radiation 104
iron-deficiency anaemia 44, 112, 289
iron supplements 10, 44, 87–8, 140
isoimmunisation 39, 289

isotretinoin 75, 76
itching 134
IUCDs (intra-uterine contraceptive
    device, coil)
  after pregnancy 256
  and conception 8
  detecting 54
  ectopic pregnancy 77, 182
  retained 217

Jacuzzi 209
jaundice 32, 263–4, 289
jogging 94
junk food 14, 84

kernicterus 263
ketones 290
kicking, fetal 139
kidneys, fetal
  damage 28, 34
  disease 59
kidneys, mothers-to-be
  damage 10
  disease 127
  stones (urinary calculi) 43, 195, 290

La Leche League 282
labour 216–17, 221–8, 290
  benefits of exercise 94
  dealing with pain 229–33
  false 221
  fetal blood sampling 69–70
  older mothers-to-be 14
  partner's involvement 156
  predicting 201
  premature see premature labour
  single mothers-to-be 172–3
  stages of 221–4
  tests during 228–9
lactose-free formula 272
Lamaze method 204, 241
laparoscopy 183, 290
laryngeal papillomas 159
laxatives 141
lead exposure 33, 104
legal questions 174–5
legs
  blood clots 184–5

cramps 48
exercises 102
swollen 5, 102, 187
waxing 210
leucorrhoea 143–4, *290*
leukaemia 47, 59
Librium 168
lifting 103, 252
lightening (dropping) 148, 215, *290*
lindane 35
linea nigra 132, *290*
listeria 179
lithium 75
lithotripsy 43
live virus vaccines 78
liver, fetal
 damage 28, 34
 disease 59
 enlarged 32
local anaesthesia 230, 231
lochia *290*
low birth weight
 anaemia 44
 cytomegalovirus 32
 herpes 160
 multiple pregnancies 111
 partner's exposure to chemicals 154
 smoking 165
 urinary tract infections 143
low blood pressure *see* hypotension
lower back pain 191, 195
L/S (lecithin/sphingomyelin) ratio 70, *290*
LSD 169
lungs, fetal
 damage 28, 34
 maturity 70, 71
lupus *see* systemic lupus erythematosus
Lyme disease 29, 34, *290*
lymphoma 47

Maalox 36, 77
magnesium sulphate 188
magnetic resonance imaging *see* MRI
mammograms 186, *290*
maple syrup urine disease 58
marijuana (hashish) 16, 168
mask of pregnancy 133, 205, *290*

massage 48, 206
maternity allowance 108
maternity bras 197
maternity certificates 105, 108
maternity clothes 146, 196
maternity girdles 194
maternity knickers 197
maternity leave 105–7, 114
maternity pay 107–8
maternity support tights 48, 102, 136, 184, 197
meconium 125–6, *290*
medicines 72
 allergies 38
 anti-depressants 137
 asthma 9, 46
 before pregnancy 3, 4, 12
 blood pressure 9
 breast feeding 273
 containing caffeine 86–7
 diarrhoea 31
 effects on fetus 75, 123
 epilepsy 46
 heartburn 36
 lupus 74
 older mothers-to-be 14
 over-the-counter (OTCs) 76–7, 167
 prescription 74, 76
 seizure 10
 thyroid 11, 74
megaloblastic anaemia 73
melanoma 47, *290*
meningitis 28, 34
meningomyelocoele 125, *290*
menstrual age *see* gestational age
menstrual cycle 6
menstruation *290*
mental retardation 32, 75, 84, 170
mercury 33, 35
mescaline 169
methimazole 75
methotrexate 75
metronidazole 158
microcephaly 32, 33, 34, 75, *291*
Micronor 257, 274
micropthalmia 123, *291*
microwaves 207, 257
midwives 24, *291*

migraine 37
milia 261
milk allergies 273
milk ducts 5, 145
  plugged 278
milk let-down 277, 281, *291*
Milk of Magnesia 36, 77, 141
mineral supplements 87–8
miscarriage 178–82, *291*
  alcohol use 166
  amniocentesis 58
  cancer treatments 47
  chorionic villus sampling 60
  cocaine use 170
  diabetes 45
  fetoscopy 60
  habitual 13, 51, 92, 180, *288*
  herpes 160
  identifying 54
  IUCDs 77
  lead exposure 33
  lupus 30, 34
  medicines 75, 76
  multiple pregnancies 111
  partner's exposure to chemicals 154
  PCBs 35
  pesticides 35
  pregnancy following 4
  rhesus negativity 39
  rubella 32
  sexual activity 151
  sickle cell anaemia 44
  smoking 165
  toxoplasmosis 31
  workplace hazards 104
missed abortion *291*
missed miscarriage 180
moles, changes in 133
monozygotic twins 110, *291*
mood swings 102, 137, 195
morning sickness 25–6, 85, 137, 142, *291*
  in partners 154
morphine 169
motor retardation 32
movement of the fetus 138–40
  big changes in 176
MRI (magnetic resonance imaging) 11,
  64

mucus plug 225, *291*
multiple pregnancies 109–15
  anaemia 44, 112
  breast feeding 275
  caesarean sections 233, 236
  exercise 92
  folic acid supplements 73
  home uterine monitoring 65
  intra-uterine growth retardation 127
  older mothers-to-be 48, 110
  sexual activity 151
  ultrasound scans 53
muscle reflex changes 187

nails, changes during pregnancy 147
names, babies' 207
nappies, cloth or disposable 267
nappy rash 261
Napratec 77
Naprasyn 76
naproxen 76
narcotics 218
National Childbirth Trust 204
natural childbirth *291*
nausea 21, 25–6, 85
neonatal death 124
neonatal maturity assessment 259
neural tube defects 59, 60, 71, *291 see
    also* anencephaly; hydrocephalus;
    spina bifida
newborns
  after birth 242
  appearance 260–2
  caring for 266–8
  car seats 219–20, 268
  effects of gonorrhoea 162
  effects of syphilis 162
  feeding 269–82
  health 262–3
  herpes 160
  jaundice 263–4
  requirements 219
  sleeping habits 265–6
  tests 258, 259
  thrush 158
  weight 258
nipples
  darkening 144

inverted 145–6
leaking 281
soreness during breast feeding 277
stimulation 151
nipple shields 277
nitrazine test 189
nodules (gum) 141
Norplant 8, 256
nose
appearance of newborns 260
bleeds 38
cleaning 267
stuffiness 38
Nurofen 76
nursing bras 197, 280–1
nutrition 80–90
before pregnancy 14–15
deficits 179, 191
for healthy teeth 142
multiple pregnancies 112
Nycopren 76
nystatin 158

obstetricians 23, *291*
private 202
occipito-posterior labour 227
Occupational Reproductive Hazards
Center 103
oedema *291*
oesophageal blockage 59
oestrogen 7
older mothers-to-be 13–14, 48–9
amniocentesis 14, 49, 56
twins 109, 110
older partners 14, 155
oligohydramnios *291*
omphalocoele 125
opioids 168–9, *291*
oral contraceptives
after pregnancy 256
before pregnancy 8
during breastfeeding 257, 274
during pregnancy 77
patchy skin 133
organic solvents 104
orgasm 149, 150, 151
osteogenesis imperfecta 58, 59
ovarian cycle *291*

over-the-counter medicines (OTCs)
76–7, 167
overweight 97
ovulation *291*
ovulatory age *see* fertilisation age
oxytocin 151, 216, 222, 224, 242, 273,
291

paediatricians *292*
private 202
pain
after childbirth 251
back 48, 95, 191, 195, 253
breast feeding 277
during exercise 95
episiotomy 238
fetal movement 140
labour 221, 229–33
leg cramps 48
pelvic 161
pubic 95
sciatic nerve 194
sexual activity 151
sides 138, 182
uterus 137
palmar erythema (red palms) 133, *292*
paracervical block *292*
paracetamol (Panadol) 27, 37, 48, 77,
138, 194, 277, 278
partners 152–6
alcohol use 154, 167
antenatal appointments 207
business trips 201
cutting umbilical cord 242
drug use 154, 155
during labour 226
equal-parenthood partnerships 155, 253
genetic counselling 52
help with breast feeding 281
herpes 161
older 14, 155
requirements for hospital 219
smoking 154, 155, 165–6
ultrasound scans 56
unmarried 174, 175
patchy skin 133
PCBs (polychlorinated biphenyls) 33,
35, 104

pelvic examinations 22, 66–7, 256
pelvic infections 182
pelvic inflammatory disease (PID) 161,
182
pelvic pain 161
penicillin 162
perinatologists 24, *292*
perineum *292*
perspiration, increase in 147
pesticide exposure 35
pethidine 169, 232
pets
accepting the baby 206–7
health risks from 31
peyote 169
phenacetin 76
phencyclidine (PCP) 169
phenobarbitone 10, 46, 188
phenylalanine 84
phenylketonuria
mothers-to-be 84
newborns 259
phenytoin 46, 75
phosphatidyl glycerol (PG) *292*
test 70
phospholipids *292*
photographs, ultrasound scans 56
phototherapy 264, *292*
physical dependence 167
physiological anaemia of pregnancy *292*
PID (pelvic inflammatory disease) 161,
182
pins and needles, pelvic 138
placenta 7, 208–9, 224, *292*
abnormalities 54, 127
problems 112, 189–92
retained 192
placenta praevia 151, 165, 189–90, 233,
292
placental abruption 48, 165, 170, 190–1,
233, *292*
plugged ducts 278
pneumonia
mothers-to-be 63
newborns 28, 34, 125, 161
pneumonitis 125, *292*
podophyllin 160
polio vaccination 78

pollution
air 123
see also environmental hazards
polyhydramnios 112
post-dates births 243–4, *292*
postmature babies 118, *292*
postnatal check ups 255–6
postnatal depression 254, *292*
postpartum blues 254, *292*
postnatal haemorrhage (postpartum
haemorrhage) 243, *292*
post term babies *see* post-dates birth
postural hypotension 41
precancerous spots 134
prednisolene 74
pre-eclampsia (toxaemia of pregnancy)
186–8, *292–3*
drug use 168, 169
exercise 92
multiple pregnancies 111
older mothers-to-be 48
pregnancy diabetes *see* gestational
diabetes
pregnancy-induced hypertension 41, 65,
289
pregnancy pillows 100
pregnancy tests 50, 183, 184
miscarriages 181
pregnancy tumours 141
premature (preterm) birth (delivery)
124, 217, *292*
anaemia 44
breech presentation 239
herpes 160
lead exposure 104
lupus 30, 34
multiple pregnancies 113
private care 202
prolonged standing 17
premature (preterm) labour 217–18
amniocentesis 58
exercise 92
home uterine monitoring 64
Lyme disease 29, 34
multiple pregnancies 112, 113
opioid use 169
placental abruption 191
sexual activity 151

trichomonal vaginitis 158
  urinary tract infections 143
prenatal care 292 *see also* antenatal care
prepared childbirth 293
preparing for pregnancy 3–4
prescription medicines 74, 76
presentation 112, 227–8, 238–40, 293
  monitoring 66
preterm babies 118
prickly heat 261
private care 202–3
progesterone 7, 181
  deficiency 179
propylthiouracil 74, 75, 293
protein intake 81, 82, 84
proteinuria 293
Prozac 74
pruritis gravidarum 134, 293
psychological dependence 167
pubic pain 95
pubic shaving 220
pubic symphysis 293
pudendal block 231, 293
pulmonary embolism 186, 293
pulmonary embolus 184–5
pulse, during exercise 15, 91–2
pyelonephritis 42, 195, 293
pyogenic granuloma 141

quantitative HCG (human chorionic
  gonadotrophin) 183
  test 50
Quellada 35
quickening 138, 293

radiation exposure 104, 178 *see also* X-
  rays
radiation therapy 293
rashes, newborns 29, 34, 261
recovery after birth 251–5
  benefits of exercise 95
red palms *see* palmar erythema
reflex assessment 259
relaxation 100
respiratory distress syndrome 70
rest 100, 253
  during work 102
restaurant food 86

retained placenta 192
Retin-A 76
Rettinova 76
rhesus factor test 4, 23, 51
rhesus negative, rhesus negativity 38–9,
  51, 259, 293
  miscarriage 181
rhesus-sensitivity *see* isoimmunisation
riding 15, 94
ritodrine 218
Roaccutane 75, 76
round ligament pain 138, 293
rubella (German measles) 34
  fetal detecting 58
  possible effects 32, 34, 104, 123
  titres 4, 23, 51
  vaccines 12, 51, 78
rupture of membranes 293 *see also*
  breaking of waters

saccharin 85
safety
  newborns, in the car 268
  newborns, at home 257
  at work 107
scans *see* CT scans; ultrasound scans
sciatic nerve pain 194
scuba diving 94
seat belts 201–2
sedatives 218
seizures 10, 187, 293
sex of fetus
  determining 54–5, 58, 71
  in vitro fertilisation 111
  miscarriage 181
  sex chromosomes 121
  and weight 258
sexual activity
  after pregnancy 256
  after water has broken 189
  during pregnancy 149–51, 152, 161,
  205
sexually transmitted diseases 293
  before pregnancy 17
  during pregnancy 157–63
shaving, pubic 220
shingles 32
shoulder presentations 239

Siamese twins *see* conjoined twins
sickle cell anaemia 11, 44, *294*
sickle cell trait *294*
sickle crisis 44, *293*
single mothers-to-be 171–5
sitting, prolonged 103
skiing 94
skin
   changes during pregnancy 5, 132–5
   dryness in newborns 261
   medicines during pregnancy 76
   problems in infants 34
skin tags 133–4, *293*
sleep
   newborns 265–6
   positions, mothers-to-be 41, 99–100
   requirements, mothers-to-be 99
smoking
   before pregnancy 3, 16
   during pregnancy 127, 164–5, 179,
     191
   by partners 154, 155, 165–6
sodium 41, 88–90, 188, *293–4*
sodium bicarbonate 36
solvents 104
sonogram, sonography *see* ultrasound
   scan
soya-based formula 272
spermicides 78
spider naevi 133
spina bifida 60, 125, *294*
   detecting 59, 71
   folic acid supplements 73
spinal block (spinal anaesthesia) 231–2,
   294
spitting up 270
spleen, enlarged 32
spontaneous abortion 178
spontaneous miscarriage *294*
sport 93–4
spots 134 *see also* acne
squinting 261
stages of labour 221–4
standing, prolonged
   leg cramps 48
   varicose veins 137
   at work 17, 101, 102
stasis 184, *294*

station *294*
   monitoring 66
stationary-bike riding 94, 194
statutory maternity pay 107–8
steroid cream 76
steroids 74, *294*
stilboestrol 75
stillbirth *294*
   cocaine use 170
   difference from miscarriage 181
   hepatitis 28, 34
   intra-uterine growth retardation 127
   partner's exposure to chemicals 154
   sickle cell anaemia 44
   syphilis 162
stomach bulges 147
stool softeners 37, 227
streptomycin 75
stress management 100
stress tests *294 see also* contraction stress
   tests
stretch marks 134–5, *294*
striae gravidarum *see* stretch marks
sudden infant death syndrome (SIDS)
   170, 266
sunbeds 209
sunlight exposure, newborns 262
sunscreens 205, 262
superficial blood clots 184
supine hypotension 41
support groups
   multiple births 115
   single parents 174
support tights *see* maternity support tights
surfactant 70, *294*
surfing 94
swelling
   ankles 102
   face 176
   feet 5, 102, 194
   fingers 176
   hands 5
   legs 5, 102, 187
   sleeping/resting position 195
swimming 94, 113, 194
symphysis pubis 147
symptoms of pregnancy 21
Synflex 76

Syntocinon 216
Syntometrine 222, 224
syphilis 17, 162, *294*
  possible effects 34, 162, 179
  test 23, 51
systemic lupus erythematosus (lupus, SLE) 29–30, 74, *294*
  before pregnancy 3, 10
  possible effects 30, 34

tattoos, removal during pregnancy 210
Tay-Sachs disease 60, 71, *294*
teeth
  babies and children 75, 76, 88
  mothers-to-be *see* dental care
telangiectasia(s) 133, *294*
tennis 94
teratogens 178, *294*
teratology 122–3, *294*
terbutaline 218
termination *see* abortion
tests
  before pregnancy 3, 4
  breaking of waters 189
  during labour 228–9
  during pregnancy 23, 50–71
  fetal 68–71
  newborns 258, 259
  older mothers-to-be 14
tetanus vaccination 79
tetracycline 75, 76, 161
tetrahydrocannabinol (THC) 168
thalassaemia 45, *294*
thalidomide 75
threatened miscarriage 180, *294*
thromboembolic disease 184–5
thrombophlebitis 184–5
thrombosis 184–6, *295*
thrush 158, *295*
thyroid
  disease 14, *295*
  hormone *295*
  panel *295*
  problems 11, 74
thyroid stimulating hormone (TSH) *295*
thyroxin 74
tiredness *see* fatigue
tobacco *see* smoking

tocolytic agents *295*
toxaemia of pregnancy *see* pre-eclampsia
toxic streptococcus A 30, *295*
toxoplasmosis 31, 34, 104, 123, 179, *295*
tranquillisers 168
transverse lie (transverse presentation) 112, *295*
travelling 199–201
tretinoin 76
trichomonal vaginitis 158, *295*
trimesters 118, 193, *295*
trimethadione 75
triplets *see* multiple pregnancies
tubal litigation 252
tubal pregnancy *see* ectopic pregnancy
twins *see* multiple pregnancies

ultrasound scans 50, 51, 52–6, 101
  Down's syndrome 54, 59, 211
  external cephalic version 240
  gauging fetal weight 119
  older mothers-to-be 14
  vaginal bleeding 177
umbilical cord *295*
  abnormalities 127
  cutting 155, 242
  dealing with stump 266
  problems 112, 128
  saving blood from 243
umbilicus *295*
underweight 97
ureters 42, *295*
urinary calculi *see* stones *under* kidney
urinary obstruction 59
urinary tract infections (UTIs) 11, 41–2, 143, 206
urination
  burning 42, 143
  frequent 5, 21, 42, 143, 206
  painful 143, 176
urine
  analysis 23, 51
  blood in 42, 43, 143
  leakage 188
  output after delivery 251
  protein in 186
  sugar in 46
uterine septum 191

uterus 221, *295*
  changes during menstrual cycle 6
  changes during pregnancy 5, 127
  home uterine monitoring 64–5
  measuring growth 147–8
  shrinkage after birth 242
UTIs *see* urinary tract infections

vaccination 78–9
vaccines 78–9, *295*
  hepatitis 28, 242
  rubella 12, 51
vacuum extraction 231, 241
vacuum extractor *295*
vagina
  blowing into 151
  inserting objects 151
vaginal bleeding 137, 176, 177, 178
  after birth 242–3
  after pregnancy 253
  avoiding sexual activity 151
  during exercise 16, 92, 95
  miscarriage 180
  multiple pregnancies 112
  older mothers-to-be 48
  placenta praevia 189–90
  placental abruption 191
vaginal discharge 143–4, 151, 158
  after pregnancy 253
vaginal infections 144, 157–8
vaginal ultrasound scan 55, 56
Valium 168
valproic acid 75
varicella (varicella-zoster) 32, 34
varicose veins 135–6, *295*
  support tights 197
vascular disease 127
vascular spiders *see* telangiectasia(s)
vegetables in diet 82–3
vena cava *296*
venereal warts *see* condyloma
  acuminatum
venous thrombosis *see* deep vein
  thrombosis
vernix 260, *296*
vertex presentation *296*
videotapes
  birth 241

ultrasound scans 56
vitamin A 12, 73
vitamin B 165
vitamin C 83, 85, 142, 165
vitamin D 73
vitamin E 73
vitamin K 73, 242
vitamin supplements 10, 72–3, 87–8
  antenatal vitamins 44, 72–3, 87–8
  before pregnancy 12
vomiting
  during pregnancy 21, 25, 26
  newborns 270
  severe 176

walking 93, 113, 194, 254
  difficulty 95
walking spinal anaesthesia 232–3
wandering eyes 261
warfarin 75, 185
warning signs 176
  after a fall 178
  after pregnancy 253
  of miscarriage 180
water, drinking
  before a scan 55–6
  during labour 226
  during pregnancy 85–6
  newborns 269
water aerobics 94
water on the brain *see* hydrocephalus
waters breaking *see* breaking of waters
water skiing 15, 94
waxing of legs 210
weaning 282
weepiness 136
weight
  fetal 119, 227
  newborns 119, 267–8
  see also low birth weight
weight gain
  low 127, 148
  multiple pregnancies 113
  normal range 97–8, 129–30, 137
weight management
  after pregnancy 254
  before pregnancy 3, 4
  during pregnancy 80, 96–8

see also dieting
Western Blot test 162–3
womb *see* uterus
working
  before pregnancy 17
  breast feeding 280
  business trips 199, 201
  during pregnancy 101–4
  employment rights 105
  maternity pay and benefits 107–8

workplace hazards 104
X chromosomes 121
X-rays 48, 63
  at work 17, 104
  dental 63, 142
  before pregnancy 3, 11

Y chromosomes 121
yeast infections *see* candidal
  vulvovaginitis; thrush